UNTANGLING THE MATERNITY CRISIS

Arguing that contemporary maternity services provide a toxic environment both in which to practise and to give birth, this book looks at how we can change this. Its aim is promoting the best possible experiences of childbearing, and confident, strengthening and loving contexts for new parenthood.

Designed to create awareness about the professional and political realities which enmesh maternity care, this inspiring volume features an in-depth and research-oriented analysis of the challenges faced by contemporary maternity services. Recognising the frequently hostile environment in which midwives practise, the contributors go on to explore its impact on women and families, as well as on midwives themselves. They then look at woman-centred and community-based ways of contributing to a much better birthing experience for all.

Important and relevant for all those with an interest in improving maternity care, this book is particularly suited to midwives – practising and student, doulas, birth educators and activists, policymakers and health service managers.

Nadine Edwards is a researcher, writer and birth educator in Edinburgh, UK.

Rosemary Mander is a midwife and Professor Emeritus at the University of Edinburgh, UK, where she was formerly Professor of Midwifery.

Jo Murphy-Lawless lectures in sociology at Trinity College Dublin's School of Nursing and Midwifery in Ireland.

UNTANGLING THE MATERNITY CRISIS

*Edited by Nadine Edwards, Rosemary Mander
and Jo Murphy-Lawless*

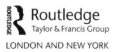
Routledge
Taylor & Francis Group

LONDON AND NEW YORK

First published 2018
by Routledge
2 Park Square, Milton Park, Abingdon, Oxon OX14 4RN

and by Routledge
711 Third Avenue, New York, NY 10017

Routledge is an imprint of the Taylor & Francis Group, an informa business

British Library Cataloguing-in-Publication Data
A catalogue record for this book is available from the British Library

Library of Congress Cataloging-in-Publication Data
Names: Edwards, Nadine Pilley, 1957- editor. | Mander, Rosemary, editor. | Murphy-Lawless, Jo, editor.
Title: Untangling the maternity crisis / edited by Nadine Edwards, Rosemary Mander, Jo Murphy-Lawless.
Description: Abingdon, Oxon ; New York, NY : Routledge, 2018. | Includes bibliographical references and index.
Identifiers: LCCN 2017040188| ISBN 9781138244207 (hardback) | ISBN 9781138244221 (pbk.) | ISBN 9781315277059 (ebook)
Subjects: | MESH: Midwifery--trends | Nurse Midwives--supply & distribution | Maternal Health Services--standards | Maternal Mortality | United Kingdom | Ireland
Classification: LCC RG950 | NLM WQ 160 | DDC 618.2--dc23
LC record available at https://lccn.loc.gov/2017040188

ISBN: 978-1-138-24420-7 (hbk)
ISBN: 978-1-138-24422-1 (pbk)
ISBN: 978-1-315-27705-9 (ebk)

Typeset in Bembo
by Fish Books Ltd.

To all birthing women and to our midwives
now and in the future

CONTENTS

ILLUSTRATIONS

Figures

Photographs

Tables

Box

CONTRIBUTORS' AFFILIATIONS

Liz Coldridge, Senior Lecturer, Psychotherapy and Counselling, University of Salford, Greater Manchester, UK

Sarah Davies, Senior Lecturer, Midwifery, University of Salford, Greater Manchester, UK

Dr Orla Donohoe, MB, former student of the Royal College of Surgeons in Ireland

Nadine Edwards, Trustee, Pregnancy and Parents Centre, Edinburgh, UK, member of the Birth Project Group

Anne-Marie Green, Documentary maker and lecturer in Journalism, Cork Institute of Technology, member of The Elephant Collective, Republic of Ireland

Kate Harris, Artistic Director of 4elements Theatre Company, Dublin, Republic of Ireland

Martina Hynan, artist and curator, member of Clare Birth Choice and The Elephant Collective, Ennis Co. Clare, Republic of Ireland

Mavis Kirkham, researcher, author and retired clinical midwife, Midwifery Professor Emerita, Sheffield Hallam University, UK

Rosemary Mander, Emeritus Professor of Midwifery, University of Edinburgh, UK, and member of the Birth Project Group

Dervla Murphy, Ireland's legendary travel writer and prolific author of more than 25 books, has been on the move across the world for over half a century, by bike, foot, donkey, mule, lorry, train, and bus. She has observed with rare humanity and increasing angst how lost we are as a species in defining our destiny, but she remains optimistic that we will find our way

Jo Murphy-Lawless, sociologist, member of the Birth Project Group and The Elephant Collective, Dublin, Republic of Ireland

Jenny Patterson, midwife, member of the Birth Project Group and PhD student, Edinburgh Napier University, UK

Helen Shallow, previous consultant midwife and Head of Midwifery, currently Midwifery Education and Policy Advisor, NMC, London, UK

Bridget Sheeran, midwife, member of The Elephant Collective, West Cork, Republic of Ireland

ACKNOWLEDGEMENTS

We would like to acknowledge the generous help of a number of wonderful people who have contributed in different ways to the completion of this book and the projects on which it is based: Abiola Adesina, Fatimah Alaya, Beverley Beech, Sara Burke, Liz Cassin, Therese Caherty, Mary Chiarella, Liz Coe, Francis Crean, Mike Edwards, Padraic Flanagan, Chris Hackforth, Julika Hudson, Stephen Hyland, Dominick Jenkins, Roisin Kavanagh, Caroline Kiernan, Michael Kivlehan, Ann Lyons, Rhona McCord, Nessa McHugh, Claire McNab, Oisín Murphy-Lawless, Siobán O'Brien-Green, Marie O'Connor, Jim O'Donnell, Eadaoin O'Sullivan, Jill Partridge, Eilish Pearce, Bruce Pilley, Ginette Pilley, Jean Robinson, Sean Rowlette, Kevin Ryan, Fleur van Leeuwen, Jeannine Webster, Sara Wickham, Vicki Williams, Lovena Jernail Wilson, and the women and midwives who have told their stories.

FOREWORD

The family experience of home birth

Dervla Murphy

At the age of 36 I had no knowledge of or theories about pregnancy and child-birth. As an only child myself, I'd never had anything to do with the human infant. So it came about that when my baby's father insisted on my booking into a private maternity home in London I didn't argue. Seemingly I needed to be in the care of an eminent obstetrician who might be presumed to deal efficiently with the first baby of an elderly mother. I did however argue when His Eminence said I must have regular check-ups for the next seven months. To me, pregnancy felt like a blissful condition and I had no intention of hanging around in London for the summer being treated as though I were diseased. Instead I took myself off to Eastern Turkey (formerly Armenia) and Kurdistan for four months. The most memorable moment of that journey was in Erzurum – Rachel's first kick.

For the last month I was 'sensible', back in London having weekly check-ups. On 3 December a brisk midwife instructed me to undress and lie on a trolley. In my ignorance, I had no suspicion of double-dealing and meekly obeyed. As some-one pushed me down a corridor the midwife informed me that I was going to have 'a little induction' – I can still hear her would-be soothing tone. Infuriated, I wriggled off the trolley – with difficulty, I then weighed fourteen instead of eleven stone. My ignorance had its limits and an induction sounded like something unnatural. I declared that my baby would be born when it was ready, retrieved my clothes and went home.

Exactly a week later, on 10 December, Rachel arrived at 3.40 a.m. At 2.20 p.m. His Eminence came on the scene; I hadn't even glimpsed him during my 27-hour labour. Having made various solemn pronouncements about my episiotomy and my varicose veins, he asked if I could somehow manage to drink half a pint of Guinness a day; evidently it's good for lactation. I thanked him for this advice, saying nothing about the crate of pint bottles of the black stuff already *in situ* under my bed by courtesy of a friend who was to become Rachel's godmother.

Most people of my generation (born 1931) were delivered at home; pregnancy didn't stimulate anxiety, giving birth was as natural as conceiving though a lot more painful. Some conceptions went wrong and there was a miscarriage, some deliveries went wrong and there was a tragedy, a dead mother and/or baby. Yet it made sense to assume that one's home was the natural birthplace, to treat the arrival of a baby as a joyous event, not a potentially dangerous medical crisis. The midwife was a familiar neighbourhood figure, pedalling by on her sturdy Raleigh with a big black bag strapped to the carrier. Soon after, we all knew about the So-and-so's latest. There must have been occasional deaths but I can recall none.

In the fullness of time I became an expectant grandmother and encountered a disquieting phenomenon: the home birth controversy. By 1995, hospital births, incorporating all sorts of hi-tech interventions, had become the norm and Rachel belonged to a dissident minority. Her mother, when introduced to the debate, overnight became a dedicated home-birther: exit authoritarian obstetricians, enter amiable midwives.

Rachel spent four mid-pregnancy months in Rwanda where her partner was helping to sort things out after the genocide – and where she was safe from testing and screening. Back in London, the pair settled into a tiny flat in Peckham which, fortuitously, placed them within the orbit of King's College Hospital's home birth unit. The antenatal classes prepared them to act as a team when labour began – at which point I realised that my own labour was the exact opposite of what it should have been. In 1968, for twenty hours, the varied midwives on duty warned me to lie still – 'Don't go past the toilet!' Then, towards the end, in the vast labour ward, my legs were raised on pulleys and my ankles shackled as though the CIA were about to begin an interrogation session. In contrast, Rachel and Andrew spent most of the twelve pre-delivery hours striding around Peckham Park, the increasing labour pains being dealt with en route. And, whereas my baby had been whisked away for four hours before I was allowed to touch her, Andrew received their child into his own hands and at once placed her on her mother's breast. And so it was when their second and third daughters arrived.

Observations of my own family scene taught me that simple, new-style home births involve only a woman not afraid of pain, a supportive, imaginative partner who has learned how to help her to cope with pain, and a reassuring midwife who by then has become a friend and mostly sits in another room, in our case chatting to the new granny and seldom intervening. I could go off course here, becoming tediously anthropological about the role of fathers; hugely supportive in Laos, harmfully interventionist in western Nepal, running far away from it all in parts of Malawi, hanging around anxiously, nearby, in central Afghanistan. But to stay with my domestic experience – it does seem to me that in our 'developed' world the father's role can be *as important* in a different way, as the midwife's. And none of the midwives I've seen in action (admittedly very few!) would dispute this.

As a new granny I became a serious (some say obsessional) advocate of home births. And it shook me to discover how many women are now too frightened even to consider a natural birth free of interventions. In such a short time, what my mother's generation took for granted had become an unacceptable risk. Even the few I've spoken with who don't want interventions do want the supposed security of a hospital setting: 'Something might go wrong…' My depictions of home births as festive occasions, suffused with the spirit of triumphant celebration, elated by the wonder of a new person in the family – none of this shifts attitudes. Nor does my scorn for the industrialised atmosphere of a maternity ward (product: babies) as something blatantly artificial, constrained by protocols and obdurate medical theories. Surely, I argue indefatigably, the happiness of an addition to the family should have a home rather than an institutional background? But no – by this stage, two or three generations have been conditioned to fear childbirth, to depend on the 'protection' of the best that the medical/chemical pain relief sciences can contrive. Repeatedly, over the past 22 years, I've seen in young women's eyes real fear – often verging on panic – at the very mention of a natural home birth. (Incidentally, should not midwives stop referring to their clients as 'patients'? A term conflating parturition and illness.)

When my third granddaughter was born in Co. Clare in 1999, I realised that Ireland's home birth scene is much harder to negotiate than Britain's. This was only partly because Rachel planned to deliver the goods some 40 miles from the nearest not very reputable hospital. Also, tiresome insurance complications proliferated and the local GP thought home births barbaric. However, a rare independent midwife was eventually tracked down and proved no less calmly efficient and companionable than our King's College Hospital friends.

By that date I had come to appreciate the significance of the 'barbaric' element. Over the years too many young women, when invited to consider a home birth, had fudged the issue by complaining that it would all be so primitive, uncivilised – lots of blood around. Yells of pain audible to the neighbours – and then it might all go wrong: a damaged baby, even a dead mother… Obviously this ties in with the ecologically calamitous aversion to towelling nappies (lots of shit around!) and with a neurotic devotion to hygiene ('Don't eat it off the floor!').

In a 2013 *AIMS Journal* editorial (vol. 25, no. 4) Vicki Williams demolishes the crazy notion that birth is inherently unsafe. As she points out,

> Healthy women usually birth healthy babies, and the biggest influence on the health of mothers and babies comes not from birth itself but from the impact of poverty in all its guises … Would nature make birth dangerous? If it really was so we would lay 1,000 eggs, not birth single babies … Why would they get regularly stuck? Nature would have done something about that, made us bigger or our babies smaller … Occasionally there are unpreventable problems, but those are the rare exception, not the rule.

Vicki Williams's brand of common sense is what this whole debate most conspicuously lacks. She continues:

Could it be that the danger and fear are largely man-made, and the modern methods of containing that danger result in a self-fulfilling prophecy? It seems clear that the three enemies of the birthing woman are poverty, poor nutrition, and the introduction and promotion of fear.

In Chapter 4 of this book Rosemary Mander notes – 'The ubiquity of women's fear of childbearing has been such that a veritable growth industry has developed and the concept has been awarded the awe-inspiring title of "tocophobia" or "tokophobia".' This pretentious label would inspire me to giggle if the growth industry from which it sprouts were not so scary, as scary as the kindred growth industries at the base of the 'rampant capitalism' pyramid: the arms industry, the food industry, the chemical industry, the agricultural industry, the tourist industry, the entertainment industry, the insurance industry, the oil industry, the tobacco industry – and so on and on, to the detriment of our own and the planet's welfare.

Jo Murphy-Lawless quotes from Marsden Wagner's *Pursuing the Birth Machine*. In 1994 the then Word Health Organization (WHO) director of maternal health wrote – 'The problem is that the birth machine is out of control'. His slightly ominous subtitle was *The search for appropriate birth technology* – but he does argue that women should be 'the principal decision-makers, alongside confident mid-wives working in community-centred maternity and perinatal services...' However, given the ubiquity of tocophobia, are women capable of making healthy decisions before they have been enabled to overcome their disability? They surely need exposure to Vicki Williams's common sense, which makes it plain that maternity hospitals are unnecessary. These should be replaced by small, well-equipped wards to care for the minority needing special treatment. Most of the generously paid obstetricians whose training predisposes them to discourage natural births are surplus to requirement. They could make themselves useful by migrating to poor countries where millions of mothers endure poverty-related complications. With the health-service funding thus made available, thousands of extra midwives could staff free-standing midwifery-led units or, better still, make the local midwife as acceptable in the average home as she was pre-birth-industry. The 2011 Birthplace Cohort Study found that 'for low-risk women having a second or subsequent baby, the most cost-effective planned place of birth was at home'.

The power of the industries listed above is so formidable that one often feels – 'What's the point of struggling, trying to go political? The monsters control all the levers...' True, on the whole. Yet in the 'developed' world public opinion, even informed and organised, can to an extent curb a monster. The health implications of cigarette smoking, once recognised and vigorously publicised by governments and modified by legislation, did bring about a massive change. Couldn't change also happen if governments came to understand that the propagation of the species is not a disease? And if they then launched a major information campaign, explaining that national health services do not have to provide expensive medical backup for one of the most basic human (and animal) activities – giving birth. Unfortunately the relevant vested interests – the birth industry as part of the general health industry – are more complex than in the tobacco case. Think Big Pharma ... plus certain subterranean relationships between *some* of the obstetric fraternity and *some* multinational purveyors of medical equipment and *some* representatives of the insurance industry. Obviously these links are not peculiar to Britain and Ireland: I've come upon them in such unlikely places as Gaza and Irkutsk.

Adding to the tangle is the risk allergy, induced by manic 'Health & Safety' regulations – another close relative of the insurance industry. Just as needless fear has been cultivated to produce obstetrics-dominated women, so the whole risk-aversion neurosis produces over-protective mothers who strive to avoid those bruises, scratches, cuts and occasional broken limbs associated with normal childhood activities.

I am not merely being facetious (or not very). From amidst the tangled politics of it all, so courageously confronted and adroitly analysed in this book, could come dramatic changes. In December 2014 a NICE report conceded: 'More women should be encouraged to give birth at midwifery-led units rather than traditional labour wards. The evidence now shows the midwife-led care is safer than hospital care for women having a straightforward, low risk, pregnancy.' As an outsider, I can't guess who or what prompted this report. Sensible people? Or people drastically short of money who saw units as an economy?

In 2011, according to a Birthplace Cohort Study from the National Perinatal Epidemiology Unit, midwife-led birth centres were available in only half of England's NHS areas and only 4 per cent of Englishwomen chose home births. Clearly it costs less to run a unit than a hospital and very much less to deliver at home where a baby's arrival requires minimal expenditure. I recall the main bought item being a wide expanse of plastic sheeting, to deal with all that blood. In our affluent world, everyone knows people with cots and pots and prams and high-chairs to be borrowed or gratefully received as gifts. And charity shops are stuffed with baby garments. But back to the central point, to tocophobia (when I've just acquired a ridiculous new word it amuses me to use it).

Jo Murphy-Lawless notes that 'birth has become absorbed into a technocratic structure which dominates the experiences and lives of women and the working lives of midwives, doing damage to both'. As this leaves so many women feeling powerless, a political campaign needs to focus on two empowering *facts* – not theories. Firstly, we have Vicki Williams's common sense statements. Secondly, we have Marsden Wagner's emphasis on the woman's right to decide for herself on a home birth or a midwifery-led unit. She doesn't need anyone's permission; she is disempowered only to the extent that she has allowed an outside authority to dominate. Or so one would like to believe. In practice, the 'technocratic structure' imprisons both mothers and midwives, as Rosemary Mander's devastating chapter so graphically reveals. In her Introduction she writes: 'A general assumption tends to be made that any fear experienced is unique to the childbearing woman because only she, obviously, experiences the actual physical pain of childbearing'. Doesn't this particular uniqueness need to be considered much more closely than it now is? Labour pains are not after all symptoms of something being wrong, which is the usual function of pain. They are proof that a happy event is in process, which explains why the memory of that agony fades so quickly. Few mothers, in times past, were deterred from having another by recollected labour pains. Yet now the industry has conditioned most women to feel that these natural pains should be avoided; that it's daft not to dodge them.

The Birth Project Group (BPG) survey of how fear affects midwives trapped within the birth industry provides enough dynamite, if it's cleverly deployed by activists, to blow up that industry. Rosemary Mander demonstrates how,

> the experience of fear is changing, that is, extending to affect others in the maternity scenario … Midwives' fear of negative stress or burnout is significant because of its potential for a direct impact on the quality of care for women.

Given our family's entirely positive encounters with midwives, I almost wept to read of their and their clients' sufferings as cogs in the 'birth machine'.

Quotes from various surveys are both heart-breaking and enraging. In 2014 Miranda Page reported that 'Midwives who worked in the larger obstetric units found the concept of uncertainty difficult to understand.' A student midwife said to Hannah Dahlen: 'It is sad but I feel more comfortable when it is all happening (induction, epidural, continuous electronic foetal monitoring) because it's what I know – normal birth frightens me.' (This reminded me of my own attempted induction.) In reply to the online question, 'What factors inhibit your ability to practise optimally?' one midwife replied: 'Staff, protocols, expectations, size of unit, the prevailing obstetric cultures of fear. Most of all, fear.'

The convergence of these obstacles creates an atmosphere in which midwives do not bring out the best in each other and many mothers become victims of obstetrics by diktat and/or the distress of those around them – the carers who should be relaxed and reassuring. Here we have one more example of the inexorable damage of 'rampant capitalism' and it is as disturbing as any other. Meanwhile, what can ordinary citizens do, politically, to improve the childbirth scene in their own communities?

We Irish have not made the most of our opportunities directly to oppose the birth industry. In August 2001 the then heads of midwifery in the three Dublin hospitals loudly protested against our rundown, out-of-date, severely overcrowded maternity hospitals. Since 2003 (or thereabouts) a multi-layered controversy (financial, theological, legal, political, sociological) has been swirling around the provision of a new so-called National Maternity Hospital (NHM) – cost £300 million. ('So-called' because it is not intended to serve all areas.) In the spring of 2017 this controversy came to the boil for reasons which need not detain us here. Its generating so much media attention, for so long, could have contributed to educating the public about the nature of the birth industry. Instead, the National Women's Council merely 'called on the government to ensure that any new maternity hospital is fully independent [of Roman Catholic control or inter-ference] and will provide the full range of reproductive services for women'. The Citizens' Assembly also disappointed by advising the State that 'all women should have access to a 20-week ultrasound scan and that maternity care should be standardised' – precisely what it should *not* be!

Very few voices pointed out that Ireland does not *need* a new maternity hospital providing 244 beds, five operating theatres and 24 delivery rooms. What it does urgently need are many more midwives and a network of small, midwife-led units set in their communities all over the country. On 23 April 2017 Justine McCarthy wrote in *The Sunday Times* of the NHM's dilapidated Victorian building 'putting babies' lives at risk'. If she reads Rosemary's Mander's chapter she will realise that babies' (and mothers') lives may also be put at risk in shiny new hospitals where overworked midwives are too often exposed to bullying by their seniors on the ward and by managers who are themselves severely stressed through underfunding. Incidentally, Justine McCarthy gave us a glimpse of the birth industry in action. 'Dr Rhona Mahony, Master of Holles Street, made the building of a modern, bespoke facility the primary mission of her seven-year mastership. She has staked her profes-sional reputation on it.'

Looking back on my own family's three joyous events, and reflecting on how *simple* everything was, it infuriates me to realise that even if women could be again brought to appreciate the value of home births there is, in Britain or Ireland, no affordable system available. We can talk of £300 million for a new maternity hospital in Dublin and we can recall the NHS calculation that 'the most cost-effective planned place of birth is at home' – but we can't join the dots because to do so would threaten the birth industry.

Some readers may feel slightly uneasy about the density of that industry's academic spin-off, as displayed in this book's References. All these scholars are of course beavering away hoping to *reform* the relevant technocratic structure. But one wonders if amassing more and more evidence, however meticulously researched and well laid out, can achieve much at this stage. Common sense indicates that for the removal of normal childbirth from the medicated zone *demolition* rather than *reform* is essential. And some of the contributors to *Untangling the Maternity Crisis: Action for Change* are already swinging the wrecking ball.

1

INTRODUCTION

A toxic culture

*Rosemary Mander, Jo Murphy-Lawless and
Nadine Edwards*

The 'usual view', the official view

In July 2017 there was an intriguing conversation to be heard on the BBC Radio 4 programme, *Woman's Hour* about the changing portrayal of motherhood in the long-running drama *The Archers*. The *Woman's Hour* presenter, Jane Garvey, played a clip dating from 1959 in which Patricia Greene as Jill Archer, the role she has played in the drama for 60 years, is discussing her second pregnancy with her fictional husband. We learn from the clip that Jill's first pregnancy, in which she carried twins, had been perfectly uncomplicated and Jill wants to give birth at home for this next baby:

> Why shouldn't I have the baby here in my own home amongst the people I love? Why should I be pushed off to a hospital … when I'm perfectly alright and healthy? It isn't as if it were my first baby or there were any compli-cations … If more women had their babies at home, there would be more beds for the women who really needed hospital care.

Garvey wonders how it came about:

> That *The Archers* thought that conversation was worthy of inclusion probably tells us that at that time there was a push clearly to get women to have children out of the home and in hospital … I wonder if the authorities asked *The Archers* to include it?

Greene observes in response: 'Nowadays it would be the reverse because we are short of midwives.' (All quotes from *Woman's Hour*, BBC Radio 4, 25th July 2017, www.bbc.co.uk/programmes/b08ylrbh).

That brief exchange encapsulates the painful contradictions which we have faced and continue to face in relation to birth and our maternity services: the suppression of a woman's decision then and now about where and how she gives birth, the erasure of her voice, the utter confusion in shifting national policies, and the impact on the professional group who should be at the heart of care-giving in pregnancy and birth: midwives. Midwives are experiencing daily the erasure of voice and skill, despite their commitment to work far differently with women, to work in equal partnership (Kirkham, 2010). They carry the terrible weight of systems which creak at best and which do not offer consistent safe care to women (Deery and Kirkham, 2007). The impact on midwives has been described thus: 'Inside their hearts are breaking' (Pezaro et al., 2015).

The predicament of the organisation and provision of maternity services in the UK and Ireland is the reason for this book. For women and for midwives, this predicament is contained in the word frequently associated with their experience of these services, 'toxic': 'toxicity' pervades the very structures of these organisations. Such a toxic system, in all its brokenness (Edwards et al., 2011), is a constant beneath what we might term the 'usual', 'widespread' or 'prevalent' view of how to offer and perhaps improve the services that are given to childbearing women and their families.

The 'usual view' is promulgated at a number of levels: by local hospitals, health boards, regional health authorities, national departments of health and the many arms-length bodies that are commissioned by the state to set policy, to monitor and to regulate, and by the state-backed organisations which are responsible for overseeing the midwifery profession as a whole (Mander and Murphy-Lawless, 2013).

These last bodies give us a glimpse of how the 'usual view' works and the language on which it relies. Inevitably in their policy documents there will be a discussion about continuing improvements; always, we are assured, based on the latest research and evidence. The Nursing and Midwifery Board of Ireland (2016) and the UK Nursing and Midwifery Council (NMC, 2016a) have both recently sought to develop new practice standards for midwives in training to improve the quality of midwifery: endeavours which might indeed form the basis for sustaining future cohorts of midwives in their day-to-day work, if much else was faced up to by the whole of the profession. These documents contain a commonly expressed official commitment to 'woman-centred care'. The phrase alone begs the question of how, if midwives are working with women, such a self-evident action must be expressed in this precise manner. In their analysis of these and similar policy statements, O'Malley-Keighran and Lohan (2016) note that in fact 'the midwife and woman' are 'largely absent as agents' while the authors endeavour to fit into the very opposite of 'woman-centred care' that is, a scientific institutional discourse' (2016: 55) which is part of the instrumental rationality organising contemporary society.

While no one can doubt the credentials and sincerity of the midwives engaged in the work of developing new standards, one needs to question what the profession is seeing and not seeing; how the 'usual view' occludes the toxicity of overladen services with care that is rushed, indifferent, unsupported, and often sub-optimal even by minimally defined clinical standards.

The immediate consequences are an increase in poorer outcomes for women, too often experienced as traumatic (Mackintosh et al., 2015; Priddis et al., 2017). Despite the abundance of evidence to support it, home birth is difficult to secure in both the UK and Ireland, due to the shortage of midwives in the former (as noted by Patricia Greene above), and the imposition of irrelevant and outdated criteria by timid health authorities in the latter. The official eagerness to render the 'Jill Archer' character of six decades ago compliant in her hospital bed has marked all our cards: the woman with no complications and a healthy pregnancy has become a statistical outlier and is considered a rarity; almost an impossibility. The definition of what constitutes 'normality' has contracted at speed so that normal birth, without all the interventions which have themselves become normalised, is very hard to achieve within a mainstream hospital setting (Downe et al., 2001; Downe 2008: ix).

The midwifery profession itself has contracted severely in the UK (Mander and Fleming, 2002); in Ireland it continues to have an almost invisible public profile, struggling against a dominant culture that valorises heavily medicalised birth (O'Malley, 2010). Policies to support women in their 'choices' with accompanying rhetoric abound. But they are not followed through by those who have budgetary and managerial power to produce concrete actions that can support midwives to work in the community where, in turn, they can support women to build better health during pregnancy to achieve optimum birth outcomes. Three local com-munity settings, amongst many, which have suffered closure in the last decade, are the community maternity unit in Montrose, Scotland; Darley Dale and Buxton in Derbyshire; and the Albany practice in London; all of these having outstanding records. In England in August 2017, a Freedom of Information request on temp-orary closures of maternity units revealed that in 2016, almost half of the NHS trusts had units that were forced to close their doors on 382 occasions to women who were in labour, with some units taking over 24 hours before they were able to reopen (Asthana, 2017). In Ireland, we have yet to get further than the two pilot midwife-led units set up in 2005 (Devane et al., 2007). Government cutbacks in both Britain and Ireland under austerity politics have made matters harder still.

Midwives are working at more than full stretch to cope with services under incredible pressure and they are leaving in increasing numbers (Dabrowski, 2017). The so-called 'recruitment and retention' problem which was identified fifteen years ago in a major research project for the Royal College of Midwives (Ball et al., 2002), at a time when government coffers were fuller, has deepened into a permanent crisis with the main reasons for abandoning the profession given as workload and staffing issues (Leversidge, 2016).

Despite these crippling realities, the 'usual view' prevails, that 'bit by bit' matters will improve. This 'usual view' is summarised in the work of Lorna Davies and her colleagues (2011: 3) who argue that the technocratic approach to birth has increased costs with little or no benefits in terms of increasing the safety of women and their babies. The organisational response to such a critique is to prepare even more guidelines, risk-assessment schedules, protocols and policies, and to seek to persuade women and service providers of the need for greater continuity of care, while disregarding the availability of those same carers. Thus, this 'usual view', operating at many different levels, even down to the management of the antenatal clinic, also seeks to persuade women that they will be safe giving birth in obstetric maternity units as opposed to other settings, such as in their own homes.

Persuading women and midwives about the 'usual view'

These efforts at persuasion are exemplified in a series of national reviews of the maternity services that have been undertaken in the different parts of Britain and Ireland. In England, the most recent of these, the 'National Maternity Review: Better Births' (NHS England, 2016: 8), assures its readers that the priority is 'personalised care, centred on the woman, her baby and her family, based around their needs and their decisions, where they have genuine choice'. In Scotland, the 'Review of Maternity and Neonatal Services in Scotland' (Scottish Government, 2017: 6) promises a 'vision' of mothers and babies being offered 'a truly family-centred, safe and compassionate approach to their care, recognising their own unique circumstances and preferences'. In Ireland, the Department of Health and Children's review panel, after reading copious amounts of international research, it tells its readers, has published its first ever maternity review (Ireland Department of Health and Children, 2016) with a similar commitment to women having 'access to safe, high quality, nationally consistent, woman-centred maternity, (ibid.: 5). Of the three, the Irish review is inadvertently the most honest: its authors state that they do not want to use terms such as 'consultant-led', let alone 'midwifery-led' because these are 'profession-centric' (ibid.: 4) whereas the emphasis should be 'on the woman'. It then pulls the rug from under the feet of Irish women, revealing that the 'choice of pathway of maternity care will be based' on a 'risk profile' of 'normal-risk', 'medium-risk' and 'high-risk,' all to be determined by the appropriate professional (ibid.: 6), thus denying a woman her agency from the outset (Wood, 2017).

Such reviews, and there have been a number in the UK over the past 25 years, have achieved little other than to fossilise the structures of the health care system and to increase resistance to any action to change organisations and services. The effectiveness of these reviews remains unmonitored and unevaluated, resulting in no understanding of their impact – or lack of it. Similarly, practitioners may also be unable to assess the effect of their practice for women and families. Instead, midwives in clinical practice are too often required to resort to strategies of obedience to those who wield power in their organisation. This is how behaviours such as 'learned helplessness' (Kirkham, 1999) manifest themselves. For those practitioners who are unable to demean themselves to descend to such a level, surreptitious high standards of skills and practice may eventually emerge in the form of working 'undercover', or 'doing good by stealth' as Mary Cronk has phrased it (Edwards, 2004: 18).

While this 'usual view' endeavours to emphasise the safety of institutional practices and routinised interventions in care, it seems that there is a reluctance to explore openly the complex and troubled background to rising maternal morbidities, or to confront the belief among both practitioners and childbearing women that the reality of breakdowns in care may lead to the ultimate childbearing tragedy – maternal death. These heart-breaking catastrophes are now attracting more, and more appropriate, attention in the London Maternity Clinical Network and in Ireland, but there remains a prevalent conviction that maternal death happens only in economically deprived settings elsewhere in the world and in history books, not in our everyday clinical world held together by the ton-load of documentation which feeds the 'usual view' and enables it to keep going in the face of all the evidence to the contrary.

This modus operandi reflects exactly the logic of the contemporary state which boasts about being modernised with its labyrinth of institutions, regulatory bodies and often outsourced services but is in disarray in its approach to the governance of health. It appears to support us in our everyday lives, yet increasingly as the neoliberal project falters, fails to do so (Mander and Murphy-Lawless, 2013). As far as birth is concerned, the 'political connectedness' which should ensure that fruitful relationship of equality that comprises the 'shared interests of the midwife and childbearing woman' (Mander and Murphy-Lawless, 2013: 185), seems almost impossible to attain under such circumstances.

Toxicity and the 'risk society'

We need to return to that word 'toxic' and discuss its relationship with what Ulrich Beck (1992) names the 'risk society' and in turn how these are linked to the 'usual view' of birth and our maternity services. The notion of a toxic culture comes in the first instance from the now decades-old environmental movement, which has consistently identified the growing avalanche of toxic conditions destroying the lived fabric of our world. These have not been accidental processes. They have arisen through the outsize might of modern science and technologies that are at the heart of modernisation and from which a major consequence is the toxic culture we now inhabit. Hofrichter (2000: 1) defines this as a culture where our 'social arrangements' have become such as to 'encourage and excuse the deterioration of the environment and human health'. This includes elements of 'chronic stress' and 'exploitative working conditions' (ibid.), important to our discussion about the maternity services.

Ulrich Beck is trenchant about this outsize might. The 'usual view' of the science and technology complex is that it is progress pure and simple which is always to be welcomed with its 'excessive potential for action' bringing expanded economic growth 'within a dominant market-centred economy' (Bauman, 1993: 211). Beck identifies 'another darker dimension' (Lash and Wynne, 1992: 2) to this complex because of the unforeseen risks which are produced. These 'hazards and insecurities … introduced by modernization itself' (Beck, 1992: 21) inevitably bring with them 'systematic and often irreversible harm' though they 'generally remain invisible' (Beck, 1992: 23). They are also differentially distributed in that those who carry the greatest burden of inequalities and those with least power may be hardest hit (ibid.: 23).

A second major problem Beck identifies is what science, with the power it has, chooses to see and what it thinks is calculable when in fact the risks its systems create are incalculable. Beck points out that scientific rationality's 'claim to be able to investigate objectively' the hazards it creates is in effect a 'house of cards of speculative assumptions' (ibid.: 29). Science will attempt to make risks technically manageable, to systematise them but only in accordance with its own knowledge base. The 'uncalculable threats' (ibid.) it creates will go uncounted, because it has no way of knowing them.

We understand these matters too well as critics of obstetric rationalities: the risks it wants to see and the risks of its own making which it refuses to countenance. For example, we have faced a major task over several decades in contesting the seemingly unassailable scientific arguments about normalising the caesarean as a way of birth (Mander, 2007). It is only relatively recently that some alternative sense has arisen within mainstream obstetric science. The WHO has stated that the liberal use of the caesarean cannot be justified and that there is insufficient evidence for the rates of caesarean birth to be as high as they are without harm accruing (WHO, 2015). However, the rates of caesareans in the UK and Ireland have yet to begin to fall dramatically in line with this newest declaration.

In this contest about caesarean birth, there are risks to a woman and her baby that have never been documented because they were not even perceived as risks (Mander, 2007). This brings us back not only to the 'usual view' but to the value system that lies behind it, which sweeps away the ethical decision-making that rightly belongs to a woman about her pregnancy and birth (Edwards, 2004, 2005). And if it is virtually impossible for a woman to make her voice heard, it is almost as hard for the midwifery manager of a badly understaffed and overworked maternity unit to raise her voice about unsafe care when the numbers of so-called elective caesareans scheduled each day by obstetricians, who sail on regardless of harm or evidence, quite simply exceed capacity.

In relation to environmental damage, the sociologists Nixon (2011) and Cock (2014) speak about a 'slow violence' which appears 'insidious, undramatic, invisible' (Cock, 2014: 113). Nixon (2011: 2) sees this as 'a violence of delayed destruction that is dispersed across time and space'.

This speaks to where we are with the predicament of our maternity services. Too often they impose conditions on women and midwives, which is exactly this insidious kind of 'slow violence' where it feels impossible to pin down how a train of events has unfolded while the damage rolls on for individuals over many years at great cost.

What this book aims to do

We have stated above that currently a 'political connectedness' between a woman and her midwife in the face of these multiple obstacles seems almost impossible, and that effective and collective action by women and midwives also appears almost impossible. We have used that word – impossible – a number of times. However, appearances can be deceiving. There are always possibilities to resist what appears a totalising order. What we explore in this book is how political connectedness can be a reality which effectively challenges the complex of problems and unequal power that we have briefly sketched out above.

In the first section, we set out the results of an online survey of midwives and student midwives about their conditions of practice. The realities are hard-hitting but they lay the basis for understanding the breadth of what needs to be done to demolish the 'usual view'.

The second section explores in detail the trauma to women and midwives that stems from the very brokenness of our current maternity system but equally shows us what can and must change at the level of institutional practice; change which can occur when midwives themselves take up the responsibility of collective dissent.

The third section discusses ways to support the energies of individual midwives under pressure and how to build a community of support for pregnant and new mothers, and then presents several political challenges that have originated in Ireland but which we argue hold important lessons for other jurisdictions in achieving an emancipatory activism around childbirth.

Finally, there is an afterword by Rosemary Mander reflecting on these arduous decades for midwives and midwifery and suggesting a sense of promise about what the future yet holds.

PART I

The Birth Project Group (BPG) survey

Introduction

Here we demonstrate certain aspects of the predicament in which maternity staff in Ireland and the UK currently find themselves. To do this we examine the situation through the eyes of midwives and student midwives endeavouring to provide the care needed by childbearing women and their babies. We use the words of the midwives and students to lay bare the difficulties which they face on a daily basis in attempting to offer the standard of care which they know only too well to be appropriate. Many of the quotations we use in this part clearly show the personal implications of the dysfunctional clinical environment in which midwives practise and students seek to be educated.

This first part of the book is based on an online survey, detailed in Chapter 2, undertaken by the Birth Project Group (BPG), which is a collaborative initiative based in Edinburgh and Dublin, comprising practising midwives, academics and birth advocates. Active since 2008, all BPG members are acutely aware of the profoundly positive value to new mothers and babies, families and the wider community, of the best possible experience of childbearing in establishing confident, strengthening and loving contexts for new parenthood. We share the view that this is consistently achieved only when the wider community is committed to protecting and supporting newly pregnant women. To do this, all those working with pregnant women and their families need support themselves, so that they can give of their best and truly be with women and their families at this crucial time. BPG activities include workshops, research and publications (BPG, 2017).

In Chapter 2, Rosemary Mander and Jenny Patterson establish the format of the survey and show the reality of midwives' and students' experiences. Chapter 3 by Orla Donohoe, recounts her experience of analysing the data and the challenging personal implications which she faced. The data which Orla discusses relate largely to the respondents' overwhelming perception of practising in a service run on a shoestring, and the wide-ranging repercussions of dire staff shortages. Rosemary Mander and her colleagues in the BPG examine, in Chapter 4, midwives' and students' anxiety both for their own careers and health, as well as the well-being of women and babies, due to the difficulties midwifery and maternity are facing. In Chapter 5, again using the BPG survey data, the aspirations of the UK regulatory statutory body (NMC) are contrasted with the real experiences of maternity staff.

Maternity is all too often regarded as a 'happy' environment in which to practise, as most babies are much-wanted and illness and death are unusual. The data discussed in this part of the book, though, reveal a very different picture, illuminating the dark side of maternity services.

2

THE BPG SURVEY

The results

Rosemary Mander and Jenny Patterson

Introduction

The plight of the National Health Service (NHS) in the UK as a political football is sadly familiar, but its longstanding instability has been aggravated by a series of health care scandals (see Chapter 5). The implications for the individual members of staff, though, have only recently been investigated by an online survey. In this chapter, after briefly outlining the method, we reflect on some of the survey's findings. Other crucial aspects of the data, such as staff shortages, midwives' fears, and the role of the statutory regulator, are addressed elsewhere in this part of the book (see Chapters 3, 4 and 5 respectively).

Probably unsurprisingly, profound concerns about staffing levels featured prominently in the midwives' and students' responses. Their heartfelt anxieties pervade much of the data and so there is difficulty distinguishing staffing problems from the other issues arising, but in discussing the findings in this chapter we seek to make this distinction.

The survey

Our research question sought to address the effect, on midwives and their practice, of the stringencies which define the recent and current health care environment. We designed an online questionnaire specifically for this survey, drawing on a Royal College of Nursing (RCN) survey (2013) in its preparation. A mixed-methods approach was used, comprising open and closed questions.

The purpose, rationale and contact details for the survey were publicised in the journal *Midwives* (Mander, 2014). Additionally, relevant social media sites were used to communicate details of the study and encourage participation. The online survey was open from September to November 2014 and was closed when no new participants were forthcoming.

For the analysis of the qualitative data, we used feminist principles of valuing agency, the individual's experiences, and achieving social change (see also Chapter 3). Specifically, we applied thematic analysis by identifying separate distinct categories in the qualitative data that manifested themselves relative to the overall emerging picture. This analysis was facilitated by the use of word clouds in the form of Wordle (Dietz, 2016). This technique was found to provide a visually meaningful way to express basic understandings of the data; it also distinctly identified initial patterns in the responses.

Midwives and midwifery students in the UK and Ireland were invited to respond confidentially to the questionnaire. A first stage self-evaluation was submitted for ethical approval, which met the required ethical considerations at this stage of the study. The initial invitation material included specific participant information and completion of the survey was taken to indicate informed consent. While respondents were assured of anonymity and confidentiality, a request was included for the contact details of those who were prepared to undertake an interview. We have discussed in detail the ethical issues raised by this survey elsewhere (BPG, 2016).

The findings and discussion

The questionnaire generated a good response from all parts of the UK and the Republic of Ireland. It was completed by 280 respondents, of whom 84.2 per cent were qualified midwives and 15.7 per cent were students. A large majority of the responses (251) were from midwives and students in the United Kingdom. The responses from the Republic of Ireland totalled 26 (9.3 per cent).

The survey showed clearly that midwives and students were all too aware of how maternity services are intended to provide high-quality care for women, as well as their babies and their families. It was clearly understood that this care is intended to be offered in a healthy, collaborative working environment. Such reasonable ideals, though, were shown by much of the data to have become unattainable within the clinical settings in which many of the respondents practised. In preparing this chapter we selected three areas which graphically illustrate the reality of their experience of practice, as recounted by the midwife and student respondents.

Support

The crucial nature of a supportive working environment for midwives was clearly demonstrated by Mavis Kirkham in her analysis of 'parallel processes' (1999). Kirkham showed that, for the childbearing woman to be able to give birth physiologically, and to care for her baby optimally, she needs to receive appropriate midwifery support. But if the midwife is to be able to provide such support she, in turn, needs to be practising in a suitably supportive environment.

In order to investigate the midwives' and students' perceptions of being supported, a number of questions about acute situations featured in the online survey. A closed question found that fewer than half of respondents, 48 per cent (n=135), felt 'very supported', with slightly more (49 per cent, n=138) feeling 'somewhat supported'. Disturbingly, though, six respondents (2.2 per cent) reported feeling unsupported. Support was further probed by an open, but focused, item:

- Please describe your feelings of being supported in acute situations. If you find some disciplines easier to approach than others, please explain.

The respondents provided a wealth of material to demonstrate their experience of the extent to which support did, or did not, happen in their clinical setting. A few midwives presented a largely positive picture of their practice:

> *All grades of staff work well together, recognising each other's' strengths and weaknesses, opportunity is made to debrief.*

Some respondents found some good support, but identified weaknesses in certain non-midwifery personnel:

> *Direct colleagues very supportive, other disciplines unsupportive.*

> *Own team members & immediate line manager are very supportive, other areas not so much.*

> *Multi-disciplinary training (skills drills) has increased support for one another, especially in difficult clinical situations. Good relationships with obstetricians and anaesthetists, slightly less with paediatricians.*

For some respondents, though, the experience of support, or the lack of it, was more complex, with the spectre of 'horizontal violence' (Leap, 1997) manifesting itself:

> *There is a culture of bullying and control from obstetricians – leading to horizontal bullying from midwives. "Good" midwives see risk everywhere, are obstetric nurses and pick on other midwives.*

> *Close colleagues are supportive as we all experience the same sort of bullying but the labour ward co-ordinators are a bloody nightmare, like spoilt brats who want everything their own way, and the obstetricians back them against the rest of the service. We are divided as a result. It is all about processing women and creating obedient production line clones instead of midwives. Women have a raw deal at every point of care. But because they have so much fucking information, they think they are somehow involved in their care, and it's all a CON.*

The converse of being supported was further explored by a closed item asking about a very different experience:

• Do you feel intimidated by other staff members in these acute situations?

While a small majority, 51 per cent (n=142), denied being intimidated, a large proportion, 41 per cent (n=115), reported feeling 'somewhat intimidated'. The number reporting feeling 'very intimidated' was disconcertingly large at 8.2 per cent (n=23).

The details of the midwives' feelings of being intimidated were probed in an open item:

• Please describe what already causes or may cause you to feel intimidated.

Some respondents demonstrated an admirable level of understanding of the stress under which personnel with particular responsibilities were functioning:

If the person in charge is snowed under.

Certain groups of midwives felt themselves to be especially vulnerable:

My interest is in low risk midwifery care ... those who feel they are experts in high risk care can be very patronising.

I feel discriminated against at times because I am part time.

Other midwives and students, though, were quite blunt in their assessment of those they regarded as their tormentors:

Scare tactics. Threats of litigation from more experienced midwives.

Bullies, shouting, threats, disciplinary action.

A supportive milieu is fundamentally important to the effective care of childbearing women. It is clearly apparent from these data that such an environment is sometimes, but certainly not universally, present. For some midwives, though, their lack of a supportive network was felt sufficiently seriously to constitute a form of bullying by various colleagues.

Standards and good practice

The professional standards of care to which UK midwives are required to adhere have been spelled out by their statutory regulator in 'The Code' (NMC, 2015). This document and its implications for midwives and other practitioners are discussed specifically in Chapter 5. The close association, though, between inadequate staffing and difficulties in maintaining a good standard of care through good midwifery practice featured prominently throughout the responses of the midwives and students.

The midwives' understanding of the nature of 'good practice' was explored in a multiple-choice item. In their responses, an overwhelming majority of the midwives and students (97.9 per cent) agreed that communication and building rapport, with both women and colleagues, is a fundamental mainstay of good practice. In the same section of the questionnaire focussing on 'good practice', an only slightly smaller proportion of respondents (93 per cent) agreed that 'Highlighting when there are concerns', which may take the form of 'whistle-blowing', is another vital aspect.

The factors which are thought to facilitate good practice were summarised in a Wordle (see Figure 2.1). This word cloud demonstrates the crucial significance of not only individual factors such as 'personal drive', but also factors inherent in the midwife's working environment. These factors, which may also be termed 'contextual', feature 'support', which has already been addressed, as well as, unsurprisingly, 'staffing'. The environmental factors also include the very human aspects of the clinical setting, in the form of 'training' and 'teamwork'.

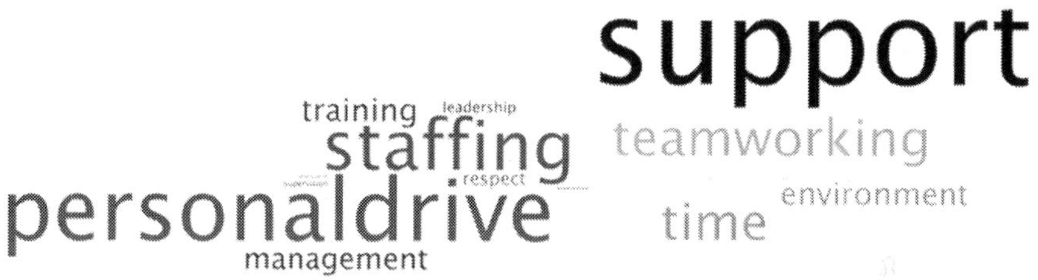

support

training leadership
staffing teamworking
personaldrive time environment
management

FIGURE 2.1 'Enables good practice'

Conversely, the factors which the respondents thought impeded good practice were scrutinised and have also been summarised in a word cloud. While the absence of some of the facilitating factors is also considered to constitute an impeding factor (a factor such as 'staffing'), many impediments may be unrelated. While it is probable that 'overwork' and [lack of] 'time' are impediments that are closely related to staffing problems, negative aspects of 'management', 'resources' and 'attitude' are prominent factors which are of quite a different order as impediments to good practice. The importance attached to these three factors is more likely to reflect organisational issues. Thus, it is likely that those who are responsible for the organisation's human functions are less than fully competent to undertake this aspect of their role.

The respondents' views on how to achieve good practice were sought using an open item:

• Please describe what enables you to achieve this good practice.

Many answers reflected issues addressed already and some were very brief, such as:

> *It doesn't happen!*
>
> *Good staffing levels.*
>
> *Time.*

The need for a more humane form of management, indicated in a Wordle (see Figure 2.2) materialised explicitly in some responses:

> *If I have done something wrong then I would like to be informed, with respect for confidentiality, not gossiped about. Sitting down with a cup of tea and discussing what happened and how it could be improved in an open and non-judgemental environment.*

In the same way, 'teamwork' was mentioned in a number of replies:

> *when midwives work as a team rather than the 'us and them' mentality between wards.*

The existence of any impediments to good practice was also sought:

• Please describe what causes you to feel hindered in achieving this good practice.

Again, management styles were the subject of much criticism:

> *archaic and unprofessional attitudes in all shop floor levels of management which then becomes acceptable behaviour amongst the lower banding staff.*

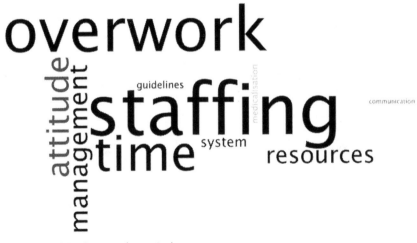

FIGURE 2.2 'Hinders good practice'

The problems that materialised in a Wordle (Figure 2.2) became more clearly apparent in the responses to this open item:

> *Staffing, poorly organised IT, badly designed notes, lack of basic resources.*

Although the midwife respondents were very clear about what constitutes good midwifery practice, many presented a dismal picture of practising in an environment which seems to prevent them from achieving these aspirations. The management of the maternity services was regarded as less than effective. The respondents considered that even quite basic human-relations activities were neglected. Thus, what may be known as the 'human resources' aspects of management that aim to foster and encourage satisfactory outcomes all round, through a healthy working environment, were deficient.

Fulfilling the role of the midwife

Closely related to the midwives' understanding of maintaining standards and achieving good practice is their perception of what constitutes the role of a midwife and, hence, their ability to achieve this role. An open question was used to explore the midwives' views as to what their role entailed:

* How would you describe the role of a midwife?

For a large proportion of respondents, this question provided an opportunity to reflect on a form of midwifery practice which may just be good, but actually verges on the idealised:

> *to be 'with woman', supporting her antenatally, intrapartumly and in the post natal period. Providing 'safe' care and ensuring that she feels like she has had good care and advice, with referrals to other parties should the need arise.*

> *autonomous practitioner, holistic, woman-centred, supportive.*

That this idyll may be less than realistic emerged in the small number of responses in which a less positive picture manifested itself:

> *The current role of the midwife is to get through the day as quickly as possible without any mishaps. Knowing the best care is not being provided.*

The questionnaire further probed the midwives' feelings about their fulfilment of this role:

* To what extent do you feel able to fulfil this role?

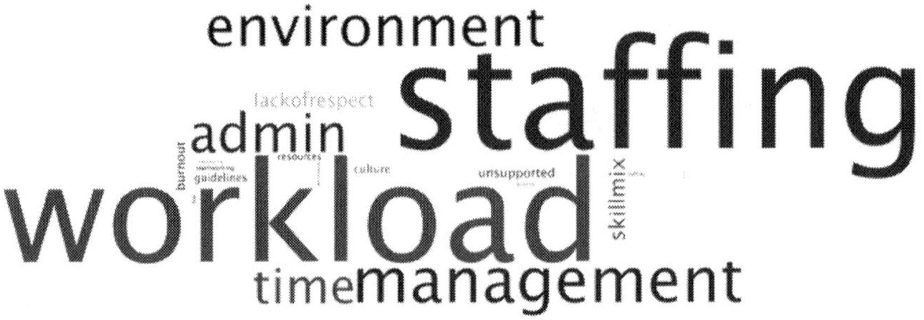

FIGURE 2.3 'Influences of fulfilling role'

A majority of respondents answered this item positively, with 57.9 per cent (n=159) checking 'Completely' or 'Mostly'. Less positive were the 118 respondents (42.5 per cent) who checked 'Somewhat', 'Hardly at all' or 'Not at all'. The factors which were thought to influence this fulfilment are summarised in a Wordle (see Figure 2.3). Yet again, 'staffing' and 'management' featured prominently, but of equal importance was the clearly not unrelated 'workload'.

The implications of the midwives' variable ability to fulfil their role were probed in an open question:

- If you feel unable to fulfil your role, what do you see as the consequences of this?

In spite of the majority of respondents having stated that they did feel able to fulfil their role (see above), many took the opportunity to answer this item. This indicates that even those midwives who were to some extent content with being able to practise appropriately, must have at least considered that achieving a complete midwifery role was under some degree of threat.

The consequences of this lack of fulfilling the role were seen to be variable:

> *Could just be some paper work not finished or completed. Can be not being able to give the breast feeding support a woman needs. But could end up being a mistake… or something missed … very near mark at times.*

It may be argued, though, that even incomplete paperwork is not necessarily a minor issue, as it may have serious repercussions for the woman's and the baby's later care, well-being and, possibly, health.

While most of the respondents considered the consequences in terms of the individual, others were able to envisage the wider effect or what may be called 'the big picture':

> *More [caesarean] sections, less breast-fed babies, more post-natal depression, declining health of the nation.*

The major focus, however, in contemplating the consequences of midwives' non-fulfilment of their role, was the implications for the childbearing woman. The possibility of errors in care was prominent:

> From the woman's [point of view], it may result in unsafe care due to mistakes etc resulting from the midwife feeling increasingly stressed and therefore not functioning as highly as possible from a cognitive perspective.

A small number of midwives were prepared to contemplate the possibility of dire outcomes for women and babies:

> unsafe and unsatisfactory care. increasing dissatisfaction with care. adverse events incl. maternal and neonatal death.

As well as such dreadful possibilities, the long-term implications for morbidity were also a source of concern:

> Inadequate education, advice and support being given to postnatal women with potential long term consequences ie unsuccessful at breast feeding and the detrimental effect to mother and baby. Unable to give the mother the benefit of my years of knowledge and experience in baby care. Also I have not got the time to spend talking with women if they wish to do so if they are concerned about their birth experience ... an opportunity to speak to a woman when she required it may prevent long term psychological and family problems.

After the contemplation of such awful prospects, the organisational problems arising may pale into insignificance, but are nevertheless realistic:

> rushed care, leading to inconsistent advice and support, bed blocking leading to the unit being diverted or closed due to lack of bed space.

A few of the midwives were prepared, and able, to articulate the harm which such infringements on the role of the midwife do to the midwife herself. Thus, the personal consequences for the staff themselves should not be overlooked:

> sometimes I go home feeling sad and that I have let women down if I haven't been able to care for them fully due to workload and staff shortages.

> I mostly achieve what I do at personal cost which cannot be sustained. Many midwives do the same and the result is "burnout". Many midwives are leaving the profession, who will support women then?

> I am leaving the NHS and will work as IM [independent midwife] or simply not work. I cannot be party to the abuse that is occurring.

These data resonate profoundly with Jenny Patterson's account of her experience of using Capacitar to support midwives for whom this personal cost is great (see Chapter 10).

Thus, these findings, relating to the inability of the midwife to undertake the role for which she has been prepared, and usually employed, are of fundamentally crucial significance. The data show clearly that the possible threat to the role of the midwife is of utmost seriousness to midwives and should be regarded with equal concern by anyone with an interest in the care of women and families. That the midwife's inability to achieve her designated role is largely due to factors in the clinical environment is obvious from the discussion of other aspects of the data.

Conclusion

The findings that have been presented and discussed in this chapter show an ominously clear picture of many midwives with the perception that they are being inhibited or thwarted in their clinical practice. Thus, they are prevented from providing for women the care which they know to be necessary and which they would be well able to provide if more congenial circumstances prevailed. The findings that we have presented here have shown a range of factors which serve to interfere with the optimal functioning, and practice, of many of the midwife and student respondents.

Of particular concern, though, appears to be the destructive interaction between two of these factors. First, the anxieties of many of the respondents about low levels of staffing are disconcertingly familiar. Second, the extent to which staff shortages interact with managerial behaviour, or the lack of it, emerges from these data. The respondents show, by articulating their anxieties, that a vicious cycle is emerging. Through this cycle the management appear to be totally ineffective in addressing the midwives' anxieties about staffing levels. While it may be unrealistic to expect managers to actually resolve the poor staffing situation, it is not unreasonable to expect that they should value, and be concerned about, the well-being of the staff who remain in practice in the clinical areas. Such valuing and concern seem to be absent from the management styles of many of the managers mentioned in this survey; thus, the human-relations functions, which are a fundamental aspect of any managerial role, were notable by their absence.

These data have shown that staffing difficulties resulting from financial stringencies, and ineffective management, possibly due to a lack of managerial experience and/or education, are serving to aggravate each other to create a downward spiral, which constitutes a vicious cycle.

3

THE BPG SURVEY

Working with the data

Orla Donohoe

After embarking on a midwifery programme, I felt privileged to be taught by Dr Jo Murphy-Lawless. Although I changed my career path to pursue medicine, we remained in contact, and fortunately we became friends through our shared passion for childbirth and women's health. Jo facilitated my participation in analysing the data from the BPG survey (see Chapter 2).

Sifting through the answers to 18 open-ended questions from 280 midwives and midwifery students was eye-opening, and frankly, very worrying. But sadly none of the answers were surprising. During my short time studying midwifery in Dublin, I encountered first-hand the concerns expressed here by midwives in the UK and Ireland.

In this chapter I will explore the most important messages and concerns I felt the midwives wanted to be conveyed. Most of them, in one way or another, related to staffing, or lack thereof.

In my analysis I employed a thematic approach as described by Bryman (2012) and Greenhalgh and Taylor (1997). Reading through the content, which ranged from single words to paragraphs, I identified common themes, and as I progressed through the data, these themes developed into sub-themes.

I extracted the statements that related to these themes, indexing the random number assigned to that participant, as well as key words that were common within the statements, and quotations that explained the main themes in detail.

New themes emerged continuously; however, the main themes were those that appeared most commonly and consistently throughout the data set.

Statements made in relation to a specific theme were grouped, making it possible to analyse the diverse range of experiences and opinions in relation to the main themes.

The data are thus interpreted and presented as themes; as Greenhalgh and Taylor (1997: 742) point out, in qualitative data, the 'results are by definition an interpretation of the data'.

Understaffing: A reflection

The most outstanding theme, and one that overarched other themes, was understaffing. It seemed to feed into an insidious chain of events that caused harm to both the women receiving care and the midwives giving care. This cycle was self-perpetuating, as we will explore below, leaving midwives despondent and at risk. The failure to implement the obvious solution, that is, adequate staffing, despite their pleas, has left midwives disillusioned and feeling voiceless:

I fear nothing will change until a catastrophe occurs – we certainly aren't being listened to

Here I attempt to make these midwives' voices heard. Repetition of phrases serves to demonstrate how I perceived the midwives to be in unison in voicing concerns about crucial problems evident to them as a result of understaffing.

Midwives, selflessly – demonstrating midwifery to be a true vocation – were primarily worried about women's safety over their own, and were willing to sacrifice their own needs to improve the care they provided to women:

Women will mostly receive good care because midwives are putting in the time but to the cost of themselves

However, many realised that this is unsustainable, ultimately leading to midwives having to choose, and some realising that survival meant leaving the profession – a sad reflection on the effect that maternity services are having on our midwives.

Understaffing: Effects on women

When asked what their main concern was when staffing was low, many midwives expressed concern regarding the standard of care delivered to women. 'Inadequate' care was a prevailing term, with midwives echoing statements that care was 'reduced to basics':

I only have time to do the basic part of the job

Inadequate care which is unacceptable

Not enough staff to provide adequate care

Unable to deliver adequate standard of care … Inadequate staffing … concern for client safety

More worrying were the number of references to 'unsafe' care and serious concerns for women's safety when staffing was low:

Care is at best inadequate and at worst, unsafe

Main concern is unsafe care for women

I believe that safety is compromised by staffing shortages

The unit is unsafe and scrapes by without harm due to the staff working their backsides off to keep the unit going

Some midwives even made reference to 'dangerous working conditions':

Some days we are running at dangerous levels it only has been luck that nothing has happened

Often dangerous situations arise from the lack of care

The standard of care given is often poor and it feels dangerous

One midwife voiced an ominous concern:

that someone will die

These worries were compounded when midwives considered the eventuality of an emergency occurring on an understaffed ward:

In emergencies low staffing can be dangerous for patients

Occasionally when staffing is stretched you wonder how you would respond if an emergency arose

That we will not be able to cope with an emergency

Staffing levels have been a concern in Ireland and the UK for some time, with evidence of critical shortages in many areas for over a decade (Dabrowski, 2016; Edwards *et al.*, 2016; INMO, 2014; Warwick, 2016).

The price of midwifery understaffing is poor quality care (Tolofari, 2014), and research in nursing settings has shown the link between low staffing and poor patient outcomes (Rafferty *et al.*, 2007; Duffield *et al.*, 2011; Jones *et al.*, 2015).

Midwives identified the lack of time they had to carry out the holistic role of midwifery, including emotional support, due to low staffing. This was linked to the potential negative impact this may have on women's mental health:

Poor birth experiences and an increase in maternal physical and emotional morbidity

Women feel anxious about birth and sometimes traumatised following it. They are not supported in becoming parents, which leads to stress and anxiety and sometimes poor mental health

Women have a raw deal at every point of care

There was a realisation by some midwives that the women were not getting the care that they expected, and midwives themselves were disappointed that the women weren't getting the care they 'deserve':

> *I can see there is simply not enough midwives to provide the care women need* [and] *deserve*

> *women and babies don't get the care they deserve and need … mistakes … substandard care*

Understaffing: Effects on midwives

The first concern of most midwives was the safety of women, and their fears were unmistakeable.

However, what became apparent was how low staffing also had serious and equally worrying adverse effects on the midwives, which made for difficult reading.

What is evident from reading the midwives' responses is how close some are to breaking point. Fear and desperation were overwhelmingly prevalent emotions expressed. It distressed me that those caring for women in the maternity setting are so troubled both by their inability to practise as they know they should and by the context in which that practice happens.

Mental illness

A striking number of midwives had concerns for their colleagues' and their own mental health as a result of low staffing. A large number of midwives referred to an unmanageable workload, reduced coping, and high levels of stress:

> *Main concern is unsafe care for women. Also staff stress levels impacting on their physical and emotional wellbeing*

> *Self & colleagues overworked leading to stress & illness*

> *Inability to cope with workload … Staff safety and health & wellbeing, short and long term*

> *I have now left frontline midwifery … I could no longer cope with being forced to deliver substandard care due to staffing levels*

> *I am exhausted from trying to provide the care which I believe women and families are entitled to expect*

More serious are the statements describing psychiatric illness due to the work-load:

We are losing brilliant midwives and doctors due to impossible workloads impacting any chance of private life. I don't know any midwife that I know well, that has not [been] or is not, on antidepressants or anti anxiety drugs

It's highly distressing, experienced staff are leaving … The staff that remain are under such stress that they are becoming ill and unable to cope

'Low staff morale' was a phrase used with worrying frequency:

Due to staffing problems, staff morale is VERY low, and most staff are afraid that they will end up on supervised practice if they are unable to care for women properly and a mistake is made

Low staff morale, stress, unsafe staffing levels

Morales low, so sickness is a real issue

Low staff morale due to feeling that we are not providing the standard of care that we would like to deliver

Morale is non-existent

Stress and low staff morale were thought to independently impact on the standard of care, and were perceived to feed back into the cycle of compromised care:

Stress and low morale of staff … leading to sub-standard and unsafe care of women

Morale being low impacts on care

And conversely:

Staff morale when it is high enables good practice

Unfortunately, stress associated with their role was not limited to their professional environment but continued to erode their personal lives, with the impact on family life being a concern for several midwives.

I go home at night worrying unable to sleep worrying what care has been missed

Sometimes I go home feeling sad and that I have let women down if I haven't been able to care for them fully due to workload and staff shortages

Burn out for the midwife and frustration resulting in lack of motivation and poor home life due to stress

Majority of midwives I work with are doing their very best to provide good care, often at significant personal sacrifice to their health, time and finances

Constant short staffing interferes with family life

Are we taking advantage of our midwives? Midwifery is a vocation for many, but it is unacceptable that our valuable healthcare providers must sacrifice so much, and that the love of their role is so much abused.

Physical illness

The mental illness experienced by some midwives eventually manifested in physical illness. Midwives experienced 'burn-out' due to low staffing, with resulting 'sickness' contributing further to low staffing when absent midwives were not replaced. Thus, extra pressure on remaining staff increased the existing stress and workload, which fed into what many described as a 'vicious cycle', ultimately resulting in the further deterioration of physical and mental health for midwives, and directly impacting on women's care:

> Burnout and sick leave is common among staff and has a knock on effect for the staff on shift

> Care given is not of highest standards, the stress levels then remain high for all working staff resulting in stress related sickness and so the cycle continues

> The worse the staffing levels are the more midwives go off sick due to stress or being run down and a vicious circle develops

> Midwives off sick due to stress and the more staff that go off the more pressure is put on the rest of us

> Sickness leads to more sickness, it just feels like a matter of time until it will be my 'turn' for a few weeks off with stress

Job-related stress and illness forced midwives to take not only sick leave, but resulted in some midwives permanently leaving the midwifery profession. This occurred among both newly qualified and experienced midwives across Ireland and the UK:

> I am leaving the trust as I can no longer support women/families/midwife colleagues without compromising my own health

> I will probably be leaving the profession at some stage soon. I have become very ill and constantly feel like a failure because I can't deal with it silently without putting my own health at risk

> I am leaving the NHS and will work as IM or simply not work. I cannot be party to the abuse that is occurring

The stress faced by midwives is only beginning to be recognised and addressed. One NHS Trust has made midwife welfare a priority, developing a 'survival' toolkit for its midwives (Pollock, 2015). While managing personal stress is important, the systematic origins of midwives' stress must be dealt with to protect them.

DISSATISFACTION

Many midwives felt dismayed that the care and support they wish to deliver cannot be achieved due to low staffing:

> *not having the time to* [do] *everything you want to do, feeling like you never do enough*

> *I cannot be the midwife I want to be*

> *It is sad to leave every shift knowing that you haven't been able to do enough, you haven't been able to provide the care that you can and knowing that it is our women and their families that suffer*

> *I also feel constantly disheartened apologising to women for things I am unable to provide during my shift. I also live in fear that the job I once loved will come to an end because I am unable to provide the standard of care women deserve.*

> *The practice–theory gap seems as wide as ever in terms of holistic care and this causes high levels of personal stress*

> *The pressure, stress and intensity of hospital shifts in particular are exhausting and it is disheartening to see missed opportunities for excellent care because there just isn't time*

The existence of a 'production line' model is untenable and causes dissatisfaction among women and midwives:

> *We work to a 'time and motion' model which would be fine in a production industry … I feel pressured to 'deal with' women rather than 'care for' them. This comes across and fuels complaints from dissatisfied service users … Overall, highly pressurised environments lead to omissions, mistakes and dissatisfaction from the women.*

> *The way the system is set up means there is no continuity for women, the midwife is as much on the conveyer belt as the women and subsequently also goes into 'survival' mode as this is how to get through another day of feeling dissatisfied with the job. Bring back traditional caseloading midwifery*

Midwives regretted that they could not provide the emotional and holistic support they believe should be constituent of midwifery care as defined by being 'with woman':

> [The midwife's role is] *broader than ensuring women's physical safety!*

As a student I have the luxury of being able to take breaks and stay to support people who need emotional care, but I see the qualified midwives unable to do this and it is so frustrating for them

As mentioned earlier, the negative psychological effects on midwives are perceived by them to feed back into a cycle of poor care. However, stress and burn-out alone may not account fully for a reduced standard of care. Demoralised staff may in fact withdraw care as a defence mechanism against 'moral distress' (Gutierrez, 2005: 236), which has resulted from the 'practice–theory gap' – the internal conflict of providing substandard care despite knowing it is substandard.

Disillusionment and frustration for not being able to provide adequate care for women may then eventually cause some midwives to leave the profession, as noted above, and by the RCM (Warwick, 2016).

I feel frustrated in my ability to do my job properly and consider leaving the profession

Good midwives are leaving the profession as they can't be the midwife they want to be due to time and staffing

It was very hard leaving my frontline job but I had always promised myself that if I did not feel I was delivering or able to deliver good care I would not continue to work

Fear, blame and raising concerns

Many of the responses, perhaps inadvertently, drew attention to the way that the individual was made to feel responsible for systematic failings, rather than the organisation of the services. Such responsibility was manifested as fear, which was an overarching emotion conveyed by some midwives at times of understaffing, and is addressed in detail in Chapter 4. When staffing is low, many midwives had similar fears:

Fear of a serious clinical incident … fear for staff burnout, fear of getting the blame for an incident that was out of my control due to lack of staff. Fear for my career

Fear is the greatest barrier to me practicing as the midwife I would like to be. If only we would all find the courage to speak out when we are understaffed

Mistakes or omissions made due to increased workload and understaffing caused some midwives to 'fear litigation', and face 'threats of litigation' and fear losing their registration:

Inadequate care for women and dangerous working conditions. I feel I am risking my registration every day

The standard of care given is often poor and it feels dangerous

Some midwives felt blamed, and 'bullied' by management into thinking that substandard care was due to incompetence rather than staffing:

I also feel bullied into believing by management that it is a lack in our ability and not a lack in the opportunity to provide good standards of care

Not being able to provide the appropriate care to the woman and her baby [when staffing is low]. *If something does go wrong, who is going to get the blame? Frontline staff!*

Raising concerns with management and senior staff regarding staffing levels and standards of care created further problems for some midwives, as they believed management would view them as incompetent for doing so:

I am also concerned for myself, in that due to a lack of time to provide an adequate and safe level of care I may come under scrutiny and my professional conduct may be questioned. I am afraid that if I raise concerns with management I will be viewed as incompetent.

If I ask for help, I have often been made to feel that I don't know what I'm doing, or am incompetent

being judged as incompetent for daring to ask for help when feel situation unsafe

As a student I don't feel I can raise concerns as at the end of my placement I need my preceptors to sign off on my competency

Many midwives who feel enabled to raise concerns feel that their worries are not being heeded:

When we are struggling and say we need more staff it isn't listened to.

I fear nothing will change until a catastrophe occurs – we certainly aren't being listened to

Others who raised concerns received 'no support or feedback', were 'told off', 'labelled as trouble makers', and 'told not to rock the boat by the ward coordinator'. Bickhoff *et al.* (2016, 2017) found in the literature that nursing students being told not to 'rock the boat' when faced with poor practice was not uncommon. If not encouraged during their training, and/or modelled in practice, one wonders how these healthcare practitioners can develop the 'moral courage' (Bickhoff *et al.*, 2017: 71) to comfortably confront poor clinical practices that cause the aforementioned 'moral distress' (Gutierrez, 2005: 236).

One also wonders when the spirit of open disclosure will become acceptable for frontline staff. If midwives are experiencing difficulty raising concerns pre-emptively about a possible adverse event, it is understandable how some might find it difficult to find the 'moral courage' to speak up when a serious incident has occurred. This wilful deliberate silencing and avoidance of critical analysis is a catastrophic strategy to adopt in healthcare, as demonstrated by the Morecambe Bay Report (Kirkup, 2015).

Portiuncula University Hospital in Ireland suffered a similar fate when staff concerns were not escalated and external management claimed not to have been made aware of the concerns raised, leading to baby deaths (Cullen, 2015).

In conclusion, my analysis of these data leads me to consider the guilt and stress experienced by midwives in understaffed areas. I question whether such reactions are conveniently and oppressively seen as individual failings, rather than being recognised as systematic, organisational and ideological failures requiring a collective, political response.

My abiding and overwhelming impressions of these findings are summarised in the words of one experienced midwife, who stated that the current level of staffing is:

An accident waiting to happen

4

THE BPG SURVEY

Fear

Rosemary Mander and BPG

Introduction

The reality of fear in the context of childbearing is so patently obvious that it barely deserves a mention. The ubiquity of women's fear of childbearing has been such that a veritable growth industry has developed and the concept has been awarded the awe-inspiring title of 'tocophobia' or 'tokophobia' (Davies, 2014).

The significance of the existence of fear in childbearing is that it has been shown to be counterproductive in the achievement of certain physiological outcomes. The crucially beneficial role of the autonomic nervous system and the secretion of oxytocin are likely to be inhibited in the presence of fear and anxiety (Uvnäs-Moberg *et al.*, 2015). In this way dystocia is likely to be aggravated during labour and the successful establishment of breastfeeding may be impeded. At the opposite end of the spectrum to fear is confidence, which facilitates physiological processes such as labour, birth and breastfeeding.

Fear in maternity has been associated with the unpredictable and unknowable course that childbearing in general, and labour in particular, is likely to follow (Morris, 2005). A general assumption tends to be made that any fear experienced is unique to the childbearing woman because only she, obviously, experiences the actual physical pain of childbearing. Thoughts about this, though, are beginning to change, which means that such an assumption is becoming less and less tenable. In this chapter we demonstrate how the experience of fear is changing, which is extending to affect others in the maternity scenario. We then go on to consider the implications of this extension for those who may be involved or affected.

Background

The significance of fear

Midwives' fear or negative stress or burn-out is significant because of its potential for direct impact on the quality of care for women (Pezaro, 2016), as the effects of the mother–midwife relationship on outcomes have been shown (Kirkham, 2010; Hunter et al., 2008). Because of the complex choreography of hormones during childbearing and early motherhood, women and babies are particularly vulnerable (Buckley, 2015).

The adverse effects of poor relationships on maternal mental health (Ayers et al., 2008; Ayers et al., 2015) mean that conditions such as post-traumatic stress disorder (PTSD) may arise from, not only *what* happened for the woman, but more likely *how* it happened. The subjective perception of how women feel they were treated or cared for is a major factor (Ayers et al., 2008; Garthus-Niegel et al., 2013; McKenzie-McHarg, 2015; Simpson and Catling, 2015) and possibly the most important factor (Harris and Ayers, 2012). Thus the effect on the woman of the midwife being stressed, burned-out or fearful is likely to be seen as part of the development of mental health problems.

The prioritisation by health services of the physical well-being of mother and baby is explicit in the Millennium Development Goal (MDG) 5 to 'Improve Maternal Health' (UN, 2015). This may be a retrograde step from the earlier WHO MDG which was stated to be 'Improving Maternal Mental Health' (WHO, 2008). This implies that maternal mental health may be less of a priority in health care services (Ayers et al., 2015).

The experience of fear

The way that midwives experience fear was the subject of a qualitative study by Hannah Dahlen and Shea Caplice (2014) in Australia. These researchers focused on the professional aspects of midwives' anxieties, but the respondents concentrated almost exclusively on the fear aroused by clinical problems. Maternal and fetal/neonatal morbidity and mortality, as well as near misses, absolutely dominated the anxieties that were articulated by the midwife respondents. Fears relating to the environment in which the midwives practised constituted only 17 per cent (n=132) of the total response. Thus, this research creates the impression of fear and anxiety being generated solely by the welfare or otherwise of the woman and baby for whom the midwife provides care. Subsequent publications by this team of researchers have made recommendations for techniques which midwives may employ to help them to address what they call the 'culture of fear' (Dahlen and Gutteridge, 2015: 98).

In the course of another qualitative study, Helen Shallow (2001) in the north of England explored the reactions of midwives to alterations to their practice environment in the form of upheavals due to certain organisational changes. Fear and anxiety featured prominently in the findings. The midwives' fears were focused on the experience of caring for women during labour and birth in a setting which was clearly highly medicalised and through which the midwives appear to have been rotated on a regular basis. The midwife participants in this study expressed significant anxiety if they considered their technical skills in providing interventive forms of care, including 'scrubbing in theatre, epidural top-ups and cardiotocograph monitoring' (Shallow, 2001: 237) were anything less than impeccable. Although Shallow alludes to the 'climate of fear' (2001: 237) her data appear to address the relationship of the individual midwife with her practice, rather than with her colleagues, managers and other disciplines.

Miranda Page (Page and Mander, 2014) built on these findings in the course of a grounded theory study involving midwives practising in a range of settings in Scotland. She moved away from the working environment, though, to investigate midwives' ability to adjust to the uncertainty, mentioned above as being inherent in childbearing, when caring for the birthing woman whose labour was being regarded as 'low risk'. Page found that the experience of fear and anxiety was more nuanced, being largely determined by the individual midwife's orientation, which she termed the 'practice philosophy' (2014: 32). Avoiding defining the midwives' being oriented to either a midwifery model or a medical model of care, Page identified the considerable variation in midwives' ability to recognise and tolerate uncertainty in a woman's labour. This is exemplified by the observation that: 'Midwives who worked in the larger obstetric units found the concept of uncertainty difficult to understand' (2014: 32).

The midwives who achieved some degree of security when practising in such technologically-determined settings did so by reducing to the absolute minimum the degree of uncertainty with which they had to cope. This minimisation was achieved by the midwife confining her practice to within her own personal comfort zone, which led inevitably to 'rigidity in practice' (Page and Mander, 2014: 32).

These findings resonate profoundly with the observation by Hannah Dahlen who reported: 'A student recently said to me, "it is sad but I feel more comfortable when it is all happening (induction, epidural, continuous electronic fetal monitoring) because it's what I know – normal birth frightens me" (2010: 160).

Thus, the midwife's fear and anxiety about the unpredictable nature of the woman's labour have been shown to be avoided to a large extent by preventing uncertainty through the imposition of medically oriented interventive practices. Whether midwives practising in less medicalised settings are in a similar position to impose their wills on those for whom they care is most unlikely. The work of Sarah Davies and Liz Coldridge (2015, see Chapter 6) emphasises the discrepancy which not only midwives, but most significantly students, encounter between their expectations of practice and the reality which they face; this has been termed 'conflicting ideologies' by Billie Hunter (2004).

It is apparent from this very brief outline of the recent literature that the focus of midwives' and researchers' attention has been the fears and anxieties engendered by the unpredictability of childbearing, particularly in relation to adverse outcomes

(Dahlen and Caplice, 2014). While some midwives have been shown to cope with such fears by the imposition of more interventive practices (Page and Mander, 2014), it has also been shown that these very interventions actually engender further fear and anxiety in midwives (Shallow, 2001). Thus the focus has been on the tasks intended to prevent harm to the woman and her baby, rather than on the people who decide upon and undertake these tasks. Because of this background, the findings relating to midwives' fears in a recent survey assume vastly greater significance.

Survey findings

An online survey by the Birth Project Group (BPG) illuminated the reality of midwives' and students' fears and that they were more deeply held and more wide-ranging than previously thought. In this chapter we consider what the midwives and students told us in their responses to the online questionnaire. The data were analysed qualitatively and quantitatively (see Chapter 3) and a preliminary account has been published elsewhere (BPG, 2015). This chapter draws largely on the qualitative data and analysis, using the actual words of the midwife and student respondents to illustrate the depth, extent and nature of their experience of being frightened. From these data we go on to draw conclusions about the potential for such fears to impact not only on the well-being of the midwife herself but also on that of the woman and baby for whom she provides care. In presenting these findings we begin by considering the more general aspects of fear before homing in on the more specific issues.

Culture

In her seminal paper, Mavis Kirkham addressed the culture of midwifery in the National Health Service in England (Kirkham, 1999). The implications of what she found to be a less than healthy working environment for midwives broke new ground in drawing attention to their working conditions. The concept of 'parallel processes' was used to show the impact of the midwife's working environment on the care which she provided. In terms of fear, though, Kirkham's emphasis focused on the organisational aspects, rather than on interpersonal relationships and how the associated behaviour may either aggravate or alleviate the midwife's anxieties.

The comments of the midwives and students responding to the BPG survey spelled out quite graphically their experience of the negative impact of culture in the maternity setting, as one midwife wrote:

> *There is a culture of fear ... I feel* [I'm] *walking on egg shells when I go to the unit, you never know what you'll walk into, there is always a frisson of fear somewhere.*

It may be said that a limited feeling of fear may be neither unhealthy nor problem-atical. This would operate in the same way that a marginal level of negative stress may actually serve to facilitate a person's functioning in some demanding circumstances. The midwife and student respondents, though, were very clear that they were in no way articulating healthy or physiological levels of fear and stress in their practice environment:

> *If we support midwives and value them, we will succeed in providing excellence. If we wear them out, stress them beyond what is reasonable – and create a culture of fear – we will pay the price in patient care.*

Thus, the respondents were prepared to look beyond their own experience of fear and to envisage its negative impact on the care which they offer, which we will consider in more detail shortly. The items in the online questionnaire included some closed questions, but one of the open items asked:

- What factors inhibit your ability to practise optimally?

In replying to this item, one midwife respondent provided a short list of inhibiting factors. She moved from the specific to listing more general factors, although her predominant focus was on interpersonal aspects: staff, protocols, expectations, size of unit, and the power of obstetrics. Most of all: fear.

The impact of obstetric colleagues on midwives' perceptions of anxiety came together in other responses, such as the midwife who mentioned:

> *the prevailing obstetric culture of fear.*

In these ways the respondents shed new light on the challenging interpersonal environment in which many midwives practise and in which many students are intended to learn.

Fear as the inability to provide appropriate care

The respondents to the BPG online survey were all too well-aware of the standard of midwifery care that they knew to be appropriate and to be expected of them. It may have been because their expectations of providing a good standard of care were so high that they were painfully explicit about the existence and depth of the gulf between these expectations and the reality of what was actually possible. That their clinical practice was only able to meet their expectations to a small extent was a major source of anxiety and fear. One midwife, as did so many, explained her current situation and looked forward pessimistically to the range of long-term outcomes, which she dreaded:

> *It is stressful because of tasks left undone, and fear has become a near-constant companion. Fear of untoward occurrences; fear of litigation; fear of burnout; fear for my health; fear of making a mistake.*

A major factor in preventing midwives and students from providing care of the standard they knew to be necessary was the staffing difficulties with which many were faced due to maternity leave, sickness absence, and limited establishments due to budgetary restrictions. For one midwife, the fear aroused by staffing problems related to a specifically sinister outcome:

I fear a serious clinical incident occurring and being blamed for something out of my control because of staff shortages.

The gulf between expectations and reality, which appears to be unbridgeable, results in omissions in care for women and their babies. Further, many respondents wrote of the extent to which shortages of staff aggravated both the gulf and the fear which it arouses.

Fear of the effects of shortages

The problem of staff shortages may be written off as little more than just a perception of a short-term problem. The extent to which this issue pervaded the midwives' and students' responses, though, contradicts such a simplistic rationalisation (Campbell, 2012; Hunter and Warren, 2014). The responses, shown in Table 4.1, to a closed item in the online questionnaire demonstrate the strength of the respondents' observations of serious shortages of midwifery staff.

TABLE 4.1 Responses to 'How often is your area fully staffed?'

All of the time	4	1.4%
Most of the time	83	30%
Frequently	48	17%
Sometimes	120	43%
Never	25	9%
Total	**280**	**100%**

As befits a professional group with a long and distinguished history and an ability to anticipate the ongoing implications of their practice, the midwife and student respondents foresaw very clearly the enduring consequences of staff shortages. Thus, the midwives and students contemplated the effects of shortages on not just themselves but also the whole profession of midwifery:

I feel constantly disheartened, apologising to women for things I am unable to provide during my shift. I also live in fear that the job I once loved will come to an end because I am unable to provide the standard of care women deserve.

The effects were considered to apply to colleagues and to unknown others as well as to the individual respondent and, as mentioned already, the midwifery service:

> It is sad to leave every shift knowing that you haven't been able to do enough and being too scared to follow up a woman due to the fear that somewhere else in the service care has fallen short. The only reason I'm still working in this environment is fear for what would happen if any more of us leave.

This latter midwife was prepared and able to contemplate the effects of fear causing greater attrition due to more staff abandoning the midwifery profession, which leads us to contemplate another even more dismal phenomenon.

The vicious cycle of fear

Fear and anxiety as causes of midwifery staff leaving the profession have already been raised and have the propensity to develop into a vicious cycle. A similar phenomenon was also suggested as operating at both an individual and an inter-personal level:

> Patient satisfaction goes down while staff stress levels go up. Fear that something – or someone – will be missed means that the increasing levels of sickness become self-perpetuating.

This cycle of fear and attrition is seen as increasing the likelihood of something going wrong in the form of an incident causing harm to a mother, a baby or possibly both. As well as such a pathological outcome to the supposedly happy and healthy process of childbearing, and the effects on the newly developing family, the midwife involved would be subject to a disciplinary process which would threaten her future in the profession.

Fear as a personal failing

In addition to the midwives and students contemplating the effects of fear and anxiety on their profession and professional lives, some considered the deeply personal effects of living and practising in fear of the difficulties which we have described already. Some midwives articulated how they thought that fear impacted adversely on their self-perception of themselves as autonomous practi-tioners. These midwives felt that they were actually being diminished by their experience of fear:

> Fear is the greatest barrier to me practising as the midwife I would like to be. If only we would all find the courage to speak out when we are understaffed and feel overwhelmed, management would need to listen.

Of course, such an experience of feeling devalued was only aggravated by the midwives' inability to resolve the situation in which they found themselves:

fear of standing out from the crowd.

The midwife's anxiety about raising her head above the parapet, about whether she is fitting in to the organisation in which she practises and how others, especially managers, judge what she does and says aggravates the pre-existing fears (Kirkham, 2007). Thus the midwife and student respondents were experiencing deeply worrying problems relating to their perceptions of themselves as autonomous human beings.

Cycle of bullying

The continuing existence of bullying in midwifery and the inability of managers to resolve the problem is a reflection of the sorry situation in many health care disciplines as well as other occupational groups. Some of the midwife respondents possessed sufficient insight into their midwifery systems to be able to identify difficulties relating to bullying among the managerial echelons:

There is a fear of bullying by managers, themselves bullied by their managers because of financial pressures.

It is apparent that the well-known phenomenon of the more senior but less capable staff member bullying a more junior and more competent colleague continues to be a source of fear and anxiety. The fact that a midwife is fearful is likely to make her more vulnerable to being bullied (Kirkham, 2007). These respondents' observations, though, demonstrate how bullying may pervade different levels of the midwifery organisation.

Discussion and conclusion

Midwifery care is essentially founded on the midwife's ability to increase women's confidence: a confidence that is likely to be sensed by her baby. The woman's confidence facilitates physiological labour and a satisfactory birth experience (Leap *et al.*, 2010). The confidence that the midwife inspires is fundamental to the woman being able to nurture her baby and to form a relationship with her child: 'It is a major part of the midwife's clinical role to treat childbearing women in ways which increase their confidence and ability to cope' (Kirkham, 1999: 737).

It is necessary to question whether and how a midwife is supposed to be able to build such confidence in the woman when she, the midwife, is experiencing the level of fear − for her job, her health and her future − that the midwives and students have described here.

This research extends Kirkham's ground-breaking work introducing the concept of 'parallel processes' to midwifery. Kirkham clearly demonstrated the way that what happens to a midwife in her supervisorial relationship may be reproduced, replicated or 'paralleled' in her clinical practice. Thus, the midwife who is not well supported by her midwifery supervisor may have difficulty in providing effective support for the women in her care.

This online survey has been able to extend Kirkham's identification of parallel processes, a phenomenon which means that people tend to behave towards others as they themselves have been treated. In this way, both positive and negative behaviour is likely to be replicated at different levels and in differing situations.

Through this research we have been able to show that parallel processes apply equally to the interpersonal aspects of the midwife's practice environment. We have shown that midwives consider that the fear arising from their experiences of poor interactions with their colleagues and other disciplines renders them less able to inspire the confidence that is necessary for a woman to labour, give birth and nurture her baby in the manner she considers appropriate. In this way, the essentially fundamental function of the midwife is being jeopardised by the health care system in which she practices. This creates the risk of bringing untold harm to the women and babies for whom the midwife should be providing safe, effective and confident care.

5

FLOORS, CEILINGS AND CELLARS

Midwives, the NMC and 'The Code'

Rosemary Mander and BPG

The Birth Project Group's online survey generated findings with important implications for the midwives' statutory regulator, the Nursing and Midwifery Council
(NMC). In this chapter we analyse these implications, reading the survey data
alongside one of the NMC's recent publications on ethical conduct in order to
demonstrate the questionable relevance of the NMC, as currently constructed, to
midwifery practice. To undertake this analysis it is necessary to examine, first, some
aspects of the background of statutory regulation in general and, second, the
situation of the NMC in particular.

General background

The origin of statutory regulation has been traced to the philanthropic beginnings
of professions (Saks, 2014). Subsequently, Mike Saks argues, changes in attitudes to
these occupational groups relegated them from being regarded as 'beneficial
harbingers of progress' to becoming agents of disempowerment (2014: 85). This
early beneficence is reflected in the archetypical legislation, the Medical Act
(HMSO, 1858); through creating a statutory register and the General Medical
Council (GMC), this act facilitated medical practitioners' upwards social mobility
in terms of their income, status, and power.

Fundamentally crucial to the Medical Act, and later legislation governing health
professions, was the concept of self-regulation; this reflected a perception of a social
contract between a profession and society, resulting in the profession's monopoly
use of its knowledge base and, hence, abundant autonomy. Saks maintains that
governments in the late-twentieth century reflected society's changing attitudes by
becoming more proactive in managing the professions. He suggests that general
management and the contract culture in the health system curtailed the power of
professions through prioritisation, target setting and the need for audit trails.

Superficially, this appears to augur greater protection of patients, instituting seemingly transparent processes to enhance accountability of and access to the professions by the public when grievances arise. However, examined from a Foucauldian perspective, these developments can be argued as mechanisms of the state seeking to prevent additional operational burdens.

Currently, reflecting the predominance of neoliberal thinking, the state has sought to offload as many responsibilities as possible, especially where health and welfare functions are pinpointed as too costly. This underpinned the Health and Social Care Act (DOH, 2012). The Act was objected to by every Royal College but paved the way for the state to shed a core responsibility: the comprehensive health care of its people in the form of the NHS. The Act broke that covenant, declaring that there was no longer a ministerial 'duty to provide' health care for all, only a 'duty to promote' health care. This opened the possibility of commercial market operations to fragment and privatise the social good of the NHS (Murphy-Lawless, 2014). As Foucault tellingly phrases it, if 'pressing and urgent events' arise, the state will move to secure first its own 'basic functioning', leading it to 'brush aside the civic, moral, and natural laws that it had previously wanted to recognize' (Foucault, 2009: 262). Such laws might have once supported very different forms of relationships with and between its citizens. In the name of neoliberal doctrines and flourishing such disingenuous phrases as efficiency, cost savings, and patient choice, the 2012 Health and Social Care Act has 'brushed aside' relationships and commitments to care, which is having a fundamentally adverse impact on maternity services (Mander and Murphy-Lawless, 2013; Murphy-Lawless, 2014). What may be the same 'game' of neoliberal governance features pastoral concerns becoming a question of 'selection and exclusion, of the sacrifice of some for the whole, of some for the state' (Foucault, 2009: 262). This is achieved by expanding the roles of 'arms' length bodies' (ALBs), government-sanctioned quangos helping the state eliminate direct points of contact where previously it had assumed responsibility for health care, including the burden of adverse events and their causes. Instead, ALBs – the NMC being an excellent example – have been created supposedly to increase the effectiveness of health care services (Mander and Murphy-Lawless, 2013: 133–135). But although ALBs have executive and regulatory functions, they are limited in scope by constraints on their remit. For example, the NMC as a statutory regulator is unable to question the complex mechanisms of the current NHS organisation, which has resulted in critical short-staffing in maternity, which might have contributed to problems of non-performance, lack of safety, and adverse events with awful outcomes. Moreover, it is hampered by the tendency common to all ALBs to behave exactly as the state does, by regarding its own continuation as its primary need. This means that the responsibility for asking precise questions and then enforcing changes is nowhere accessible for the ordinary person. It leaves virtually powerless those affected by some catastrophic incident. This outcome is welcomed by the neoliberal state, which is far from neutral and even-handed in its actions towards ordinary people. Thus, despite the NMC having regulatory potential, it exemplifies Wendy Brown's over-regulated, over-administered, under-resourced society (2001).

Major health care scandals have reinforced the perceived need for more robust external statutory regulation with such well-publicised *causes célèbres*, including the Bristol Royal Infirmary paediatric heart surgery and the Alder Hey tissue removal outrages (Allsop and Saks, 2002) as well as the Beverley Allitt case (DoH, 1994). Still more widely publicised was the case of the general practitioner and serial killer Harold Shipman who was found to have murdered an indeterminate number of patients (Smith, 2002–2005). One major finding of the Shipman enquiry was the paltry standard of oversight of, in that case, medical professionals. This criticism was applied equally to other statutory regulatory bodies and, as a result, a 'super regulator', the Council for the Regulation of Health Care Professionals (CRHP), emerged. The CRHP was to become the Council for Healthcare Regulatory Excellence (CHRE), which morphed into the Professional Standards Authority for Health and Social Care (PSA, 2016). Through these bodies the professions' highly prized self-regulation was becoming threatened to the point of vanishing (Hurwitz 2008).

The reality of statutory regulation has traditionally, according to Mary Chiarella and Jill White (2013), been manifested in four distinct elements which may be interrelated. First, entry into the profession and practitioner status are controlled by registration, which is closely associated with the would-be registrant having completed the second element: a validated or accredited educational programme. After these initial barriers, the third element, the implementation of professional advice and standards, assumes greater significance; closely linked to possible deviations from these is the fourth element, the management of complaints. Chiarella and White consider that complaints result from 'a lack of competence in the performance of their professional role; an impairment issue such as a physical or mental illness disability or an addiction to drugs or alcohol or a conduct matter' (2013: 1273). Whether this list is comprehensive and the risk of further action by the regulatory body are issues to which we will return. The professional advice and standards decreed by the statutory regulatory bodies create the 'floors and ceilings' (Chiarella 1995: 68), being the lowest acceptable and highest realistically envisaged standards. It is in the space between these levels that the competent practitioner or professional is expected to practise.

The UK Nursing and Midwifery Council (NMC)

Following the Nurses, Midwives and Health Visitors Act (1979), the three Central Midwives Boards ceased to exist when the United Kingdom Central Council (UKCC) was formed in 1983. Thus ended a period of formalised medical domination of midwifery (Fleming, 2002), which was only to be supplanted with domination by nursing. The UKCC was just one of a multitude of regulatory bodies spanning the four countries of the UK and it was replaced by the NMC in 2002. The dysfunctional nature of the NMC soon became apparent, though, attracting the attention of a review by the (then) CHRE (2012). The dire state of the NMC as a statutory regulatory body, which has been addressed in detail elsewhere (Mander, 2016), was such that CHRE recommended 15 changes: in leadership, culture, finance and operational management.

The NMC probably considered that it had narrowly escaped the backlash of the largely medical scandals mentioned above. This was until the series of calamities and misrepresentations that led to the Morecambe Bay Investigation (Kirkup, 2015) showed that midwifery services are far from immune to the problems identified elsewhere, such as in Mid-Staffordshire (Francis Report, 2013). The NMC's knee-jerk reaction to Kirkup took the form of the publication of 'The Code' (2015), which comprises a response to the scathing condemnation of the CHRE review (2012) while simultaneously seeking to address still more recent censure from the Francis report (Francis, 2013). Thus, the not-unrelated problems of a dysfunctional statutory regulatory body, together with a profession perceived to be disengaged from its patients and clients, were to be resolved with one apparently simple booklet, effectively killing two birds with one stone.

Thus, the publication of 'The Code' represents an attempt by the NMC to achieve the third element of the statutory body typology outlined by Chiarella and White (2013), that is, the provision of professional advice and standards. In order to do this 'The Code' employs a positive perspective, emphasising the near-universal adherence to the non-negotiable and non-discretionary standards that it outlines. Never far behind the carrot of this upbeat orientation, though, always lurks the stick of the threat practitioners are all too aware of – that is, disciplinary action, removal from the register and termination of the person's livelihood (NMC, 2015: 2). It is this ever-present threat of disciplinary action which Chiarella and White (2013) chose not to include in their admirable analysis of the elements of statutory regulation, mentioned above.

'The Code' may be regarded as an example of Mary Chiarella's 'floors and ceilings' approach (1995) to standard setting. This approach presents a 'floor' or minimum standard below which no competent and conscientious practitioner should ever allow her practice to deteriorate. The 'ceilings', on the other hand, provide ambitious ideals to which every practitioner should and would, in a perfect world, aspire. In our examination of the data from the online survey, we should bear in mind these two boundaries and how they relate to the experiences of the midwife and student respondents.

Findings and comparisons

In this section we consider some of the requirements of 'The Code' and the extent to which these demands correspond to the experiences of the midwife and student respondents.

Priorities

Standard setting inevitably requires the establishment of priorities and the NMC does this in the form of a response to the scathing criticisms of practitioners' pathological disengagement in the Francis report (Francis, 2013). This response is the need to 'Prioritise People' (p. 4), which equates with Francis's problematic (lack of) 'engagement'. The NMC defines this concept as 'Treat people as individuals and uphold their dignity' (p. 4) and this apparently basic requirement is elucidated in terms of:

- 1.2. Make sure you deliver the fundamentals of care effectively

Their difficulty in providing even such a basic, elemental form of care was frequently articulated by respondents to the survey. This difficulty pertained most when, as not uncommonly applied, staffing was low:

> [I fear] *That I will not have the time to care for the women and families adequately and safely.*

Immediacy

The perception of a lack of sufficient time to provide appropriate care, as mentioned by one midwife respondent, contrasts markedly with the requirements of 'The Code':

- 1.4. Make sure that any treatment, assistance or care for which you are responsible is delivered without undue delay

The midwives' and students' difficulties with managing their time, and providing care as a matter of urgency, were a frequently recurring theme and a problem which does not seem to be recognised by the NMC. The danger is that not only are urgently necessary interventions likely to be delayed but they are at risk of being completely omitted, with adverse consequences for those involved:

> *When it is busy on the post-natal ward, it is not possible to spend time providing women with information to support them in feeding and caring for their babies. This may have a negative effect on breast-feeding rates.*

Best practice

The standard of midwifery interventions is required by 'The Code' to be the highest in order to meet the benchmarks set by research-based evidence and to accord with best-practice guidelines: 'You assess need and deliver or advise on treatment ... on the basis of the best evidence available and best practice' (p. 7).

Midwives' and students' need to adopt 'best practice' tended to be viewed through the lens of staffing problems and the limited time available to provide care. Inevitably, in such situations the spectre of safety manifested itself:

[concerns about] *safety of patients being treated by over-tired staff. No time to provide the care you really want to give.*

Midwife and student respondents were all too clear that they were very well aware of what best practice comprised but they were seriously remorseful that they were prevented from achieving it by the circumstances of their practice over which they had no control. Additionally, in the context of best-practice guidelines, many respondents were scornful of the attitudes of those alongside whom they practised:

work place traditions that are not in guidelines eg. 'that's what we do here'.

As well as being required to adopt the local practices, some midwives were scathing of policies which they knew to have fallen behind the recommendations of current research evidence. As a result, midwives reported being required to be more 'flexible' in their interpretation of policies:

Midwives appear to be very fearful. We are encouraged to "bend" guidelines rather than actively challenge those that are clearly outdated and inappropriate.

Safety

According to 'The Code', the preservation of safety (p. 11) applies to the welfare of not only the 'patient' but also the general public. But the responses show that for many midwives even ensuring the safety of the women and their babies presents a serious source of anxiety:

my concerns are around safety and quality of care for women and babies, also around quality of working environment.

unsafe practice, things getting missed because we are rushing to provide basic care. Women not having the help and support to be equipped with the skills needed to be parents.

Perhaps even more disconcertingly, 'The Code' does not seem to recognise the implications of the midwife's need to preserve safety – and of the consequences and effects when the midwife is prevented from achieving this basic standard:

I go home at night worrying unable to sleep, worrying what care has been missed and often phone the unit in the middle of the night as I remember things that have been missed that's not always apparent at handover when everything that has happened during the day is still a muddle in my head. I also feel constantly disheartened apologising to women all shift for things I am unable to provide during my shift. I also live in fear that the job I once loved will come to an end.

It may be that the NMC's concern for the safety of patients and of the public may need to be extended to include the safety of the practitioners themselves.

Candour

The need for the practitioner to be candid in raising concerns and escalating them is emphasised in 'The Code' as 'the duty of candour' (p. 11). Knowledge and observation of the relevant legislation and policies is regarded as crucial in the care of those who are vulnerable. The midwives were familiar with these procedures and some seemed content with the functioning of this system. There was a consistent trend in the data, however, for midwives to report that the system of raising concerns was not utilised appropriately:

> *There is a very clear method for raising a concern which is an 'incident form'. However since it is now online it takes approximately 20 minutes to complete without interruption. If the situation is complicated or unusual it can take approx 40 minutes to complete. So when a member of staff has reached the end of her 12/13 hr shift and is already late she often is unable to do so. Even if she leaves it for the next shift she may then forget or that shift is too busy again and so it doesn't get filled in. ... When we recorded them in a book it took only a few minutes and probably 95 percent were completed. Now however I believe that only about 20–30 percent get recorded.*

From those who had used the system there were further reports of its ineffectiveness:

> *I do it and fill in the forms but nothing gets done, hence why Morecambe Bay could happen anywhere.*

While, as mentioned already, 'The Code' encourages the protection of the 'vulnerable' (p. 3), it fails to elucidate who these vulnerable people actually are. The NMC would have us believe that this label refers only to the 'patient and public'. It is necessary to consider, however, whether certain practitioners should also be included in this category:

> *The risk midwife is always encouraging us to report incidents, then she does a monthly report on it and it's nearly always the midwife who gets the rap. The comments usually say the midwife has been warned about her practice and 'I will ask the consultant to discuss with the reg or SHO'. Which basically means nothing. Also people that enter incidents are usually thought of as snitches or they enter incidents about people they don't like or because they are cross about what happened. Rather than wanting to avoid it happening again. I personally enter quite a few incidents because I want to see change, but others think I am a trouble maker.*

Harmony

With the welfare of patients and the public in mind, 'The Code' indicates that the importance of cooperative functioning (p. 8) is second only to clear communication. In response to an item questioning the midwife's ability to fulfil her role, some issues relating to harmonious interdisciplinary cooperation were raised:

> *staffing levels – some obstetric intervention is defensive and not always in the best interest of the women and in being the women's advocate there is sometimes conflict between midwifery and obstetric opinions. Also … the risk management is very critical and undermines confidence in upholding midwifery autonomy.*

It appears that such harmonious cooperation may be sought by midwives, but that their endeavours are too one-sided to achieve success.

The variability in medical support emerged from one midwife based in the community:

> *Anaesthetists are more supportive and paediatricians the least – understandable as some of them think that birth at home is a form of child abuse.*

A very welcome point, which 'The Code' includes in the section on cooperative functioning, relates to collegial support (p 8): 'be supportive of colleagues who are encountering health or performance problems. However, this support must never compromise or be at the expense of patient or public safety' (Section 8.7).

A small number of midwives' experiences corresponded with 'The Code's' requirements:

> *We have a good team and reflect practice issues supportively.*

There were many others, though, who were less able to reflect such support. In response to an item about intimidation a midwife retorted:

> *bullying, harassment, unreasonable demands and expectations from senior staff, lack of regard, trust in and support of staff resulting in apathy, demotivation and HATING work, sick leave rates go up production goes down, nobody interested in anything but covering their own back.*

The role of the midwife in facilitating harmonious interdisciplinary functioning appears to be even more difficult currently than when Jenny Kitzinger and her colleagues undertook their insightful research in 1990 (Kitzinger *et al.*, 1990).

Discussion and conclusion

From the sample of findings of the BPG online survey which we have discussed, it is clear that an addition is necessary to Chiarella and White's typology of elements of statutory regulation (2013: 1273). That unmet standards and hence complaints may be associated with various factors which they listed (see General background, above) is undeniable. To their list, though, must be added aspects of the clinical environment that are uncontrollable by even the most able midwife; these aspects would include, for example, the lack of suitably qualified staff.

The findings discussed here clearly demonstrate the lack of correspondence between 'The Code' and the reality of midwifery practice in the twenty-first century. The role of the statutory regulatory body in setting standards for the members of a professional group is clearly important and is constantly under review (NMC, 2016b). Establishing standards in terms of the floors and ceilings between which practitioners act and are able to function to the benefit of clients and patients is likely to be helpful, particularly to those who are newly qualified.

The depiction of high standards as ceilings in 'The Code' presents the clinical midwife with aims, probably most relevant to an ideal world, to which she is able to aspire. That such stratospherically high standards be demanded of the practising midwife represents a departure from the reality of the clinical environment, which is doomed to lead to failure of compliance. The floors of standard setting would represent a more realistic view of the world of the twenty-first-century midwife, but floors are absent from 'The Code'.

The findings that we have discussed in this chapter portray the reality of midwifery practice as barely reaching the level of the floor. The midwives and students who responded to our online survey report their perceptions of practising in terms of the standards which they are able to offer: below the floor in some kind of sub-basement or cellar.

Further, 'The Code' is presented as requiring absolutes in terms of setting priorities, acting immediately, demonstrating best practice, ensuring safety and being candid. Such unequivocal requirements may not be achievable in the milieu of the modern health care system and do not allow for the judgement which is a characteristic of the educated professional. Clinical judgement should be an option for midwives, as it is for other health professionals (Kienle and Kiene, 2011).

For these reasons we argue that, for the floors and ceilings to be realistic, acceptable and effective, it is crucial for the standard setters to possess an accurate impression of the actuality of both the practice of (in this case) the clinical midwife and the context of midwifery practice. This online survey has demonstrated that even such basic prerequisites are lacking in the case of the NMC.

PART II

Understanding traumatic experiences for women, midwives, families and the wider community

Introduction

The following chapters, by authors in different settings and geographical locations in the UK, all speak of the painful struggle that women, student midwives and midwives are forced to engage in while birthing their babies, or during their day-to-day practice. Using strikingly similar language, women, student midwives and midwives describe the 'irresistibility' and 'conveyor belt' nature of current maternity services in which their agency is undermined.

Women and midwives are unable to form the protective trusting relationships in a system that has adopted a business model based on outmoded factory principles that prioritise tasks and rules over nurturing and caring. This is wholly inappropriate for maternity services and results in unbearable emotional and physical costs to mothers, student midwives and midwives, as well as untenable financial costs to the state.

Women's, student midwives' and midwives' spirits and aspirations are 'broken' by the pressures to conform and 'fit in' and trapped by the corrosive standardisation, fear and blame that pervade current maternity care. It is horrifying to 'see' how the long fingers of neoliberalism increasingly stretch out and take hold of our day-to-day lives and the devastating consequences this has for maternity care on women, student midwives and midwives.

This system itself is broken. It can only change if trusting relationships between women, student midwives and midwives are enabled to flourish. As the authors point out, the policies for maternity care in the UK recommend that maternity services should be based around continuity of carer, and we already have examples of this working stunningly well (Homer *et al.*, 2017). Resources, education, training, community and workforce engagement and support need to be carefully put in place in order for the new model of care to be sustainable and responsive to good evidence and expressed community needs.

6

TRAUMA EXPERIENCED BY STUDENT MIDWIVES

Sarah Davies and Liz Coldridge

Introduction

Research has recently focused on the extent to which midwives suffer traumatic stress as a result of the work they do (Leinweber *et al.*, 2017b; Pezaro, 2016; Beck *et al.*, 2015; Sheen *et al.*, 2015; Rice and Warland, 2013). Witnessing traumatic events in childbirth, and working in a negative organisational culture (where there are staff shortages, conflicting ideologies, and lack of support for staff) have both been implicated in findings of a high level of emotional distress amongst midwives. Midwives are also more likely to report work-related distress than other healthcare professionals (Griffiths, 2016). The highly empathetic relationship between midwives and women is seen as an important element in midwives' work-related trauma (Rice and Warland, 2013). In a large UK-based survey of midwives who had experienced traumatic birth events, a third of the sample reported clinically relevant post-traumatic stress symptoms (Sheen *et al.*, 2015); while an online survey of Australian midwives found that 33 per cent of the respondents met the criteria for post-traumatic stress disorder (PTSD) and that those midwives were four times more likely than others to express an intention to leave midwifery (Leinweber *et al.*, 2017b).

Students' experiences during their course shape their professional attitudes (Jameton, 1984), and traumatic experiences may have enduring adverse effects, including a high attrition rate from the profession. In consideration of this it is important to explore how student midwives might be affected by trauma and how best to support them. With this in mind we conducted the first study of the traumatic experiences of student midwives (Davies and Coldridge, 2015; Coldridge and Davies, 2017). We interviewed 11 student midwives in the second and third years of their undergraduate course in one university in the North West of England. The method we used was interpretive phenomenological analysis (IPA) in order to allow for open exploration of the topic (Smith and Osborn, 2008). After conducting thematic analysis, we concluded that the student midwife inhabits a uniquely vulnerable position in what one described as the 'no man's land' of hospital practice. Five main themes emerged from the analysis. 'Wearing your blues' depicted the 'bleak' landscape of practice and students' enculturation into the profession. 'No man's land' was concerned with the traumatic tensions in the student role and exploring their role in the existential space between the woman and the qualified midwives. Three further themes described the experience of being in emergency or unforeseen events in practice and how they coped with them ('Get the red box!', 'The aftermath' and 'Learning to cope').

To avoid prejudging what students found traumatic we did not set criteria for trauma. For several students, what they found distressing was not necessarily a specific traumatic event but the environment in which they were working, and their own feelings of powerlessness within it; while others recounted emergency situations which were made more traumatic by taking place in this difficult environment. This chapter will explore some aspects of the themes in the light of the current crisis in UK maternity services and what needs to change.

'Wearing your blues'

The phrase 'wearing your blues' captures students' concept of the midwifery role in two ways. The blue uniform symbolises the responsibilities carried by the midwife, while the 'blues' also depicts their sense of disappointment with the realities of the role. This sense of disappointment or 'shattered fairy tale' has been identified in research exploring the role of newly qualified midwives (NQMs) too, where the 'idealised fiction' of midwifery disappeared as they qualified and began to practice (Reynolds et al., 2014: 664).

Similarly, Carolan (2011) noted in a longitudinal Australian study that student midwives begin their education with a powerful motivation to support childbearing women and well-defined ideas about what constitutes a 'good midwife'. She found that as students progressed through the course their views became 'more aligned' with those of qualified midwives, but nonetheless concluded even at the end of the course that the students' 'intense passion and enthusiasm for midwifery practice may make them vulnerable to disappointment with the profession' (Carolan, 2013: 115). She refers to this enthusiasm as 'somewhat extreme' (2013: 120), inferring that students need to adapt their unrealistic expectations to avoid disillusionment, and in order to minimise attrition from the workforce.

However, students' passionately held ideals are consonant with the rhetoric about maternity care that has informed UK government policy since 1993 – from the 'choice, continuity and control' of *Changing Childbirth* (DoH, 1993) to the most recent maternity services review in England: 'Personalised care, centred on the woman, her baby and her family, based around their needs and their decisions, where they have genuine choice, informed by unbiased information' (NHS England, 2016: 7).

The Scottish Government (2017) maternity services review similarly focuses on the central importance of the mother-midwife relationship, recommending that services be reconfigured to ensure continuity of the midwifery carer. Indeed, the notion of holistic partnership working with women is further reiterated in the curricula of Higher Education institutions through the Nursing and Midwifery Council midwifery competencies (NMC, 2009) and by midwifery professional bodies both national and international (RCM, 2016a; ICM, 2017). The vision is alive and kicking in the rhetoric of care but contrasts starkly with the protocolised care that students in our study witnessed and experienced in obstetric units. Students talked of striving to be the 'ideal' midwife in an environment where that was difficult, if not impossible:

> *I would strive not to be that institutionalised midwife, you know, if there was an option that wasn't so difficult, where you could be the midwife where you're on your hands and knees and that woman looks in your eyes and she can **see** how much you care!*

Struggling with the contradictions between the 'with-woman' philosophy and the constraints of the hospital system is not peculiar to the situation of students but has been noted in NQMs and team-based hospital midwives (Hunter, 2004), as well as implicated as a major factor in midwives' decisions to leave the profession (Curtis *et al.*, 2006). As Kirkham (2017c) observes: '… NHS midwives are torn apart. Their leaders speak the rhetoric of midwifery while clinical midwives work within the reality of a service aiming for maximum efficiency'. The drive to achieve ever-greater 'efficiencies' (such as centralisation of obstetric units, minimum staffing levels and midwives being moved at short notice by managers) is part and parcel of the marketisation and commodification of the NHS set in train in the UK by the Conservatives in 1979 and further developed and entrenched by successive governments (Mander and Murphy-Lawless, 2013). Reiger and Lane (2013: 133) point out: 'Provision of personalised, continuous care focused on "well women" is now central to midwifery identity and work ideals, but it remains difficult in hospital contexts shaped by increased demand and by neoliberal policies'. Echoing Walsh (2006: 1331) who described the environment as an 'assembly line', students suggested that psychological support for women was seen as a dispensable extra:

> *it's just like a conveyor belt getting people in and getting people out just doing the basic care rather than giving that extra care that they might need to, they might have a nice healthy baby but they might have wanted more like the emotional side or the psychological support that might have meant more to them than just a good outcome.*

The tension between their deeply held ideals and the realities of working in a busy obstetric unit was experienced by the students as deeply distressing:

Everything's standard practice where the woman almost becomes invisible and I think those sorts of behaviours are so deeply entrenched it becomes quite distressing if not traumatic ... I'm not sure about the word traumatic, I think, but certainly deeply distressing to see women treated in that way I think and sort of processed through a system...

Another perspective on the commodification of care, and the damage it does to both patients and carers is offered by Rizq (2012). From a psychotherapeutic perspective she argues that the privileging of attention to targets and protocols acts to reduce feelings of empathy, diminishing the caring role and indeed resulting in what she terms 'a perversion of care'. Furthermore, the focus on risk governance and protocols serves to disavow, or mask, the anxiety of recognising the limits to our capacity to care in such environments (Rizq, 2012: 9).

Students found it distressing when women's needs were not listened to and when women did not receive the care they knew to be appropriate. Witnessing poor practice had profound consequences not just for the women but also for students and qualified midwives:

it broke my midwifery spirit. To me it was just a big processing plant

and:

I have known people, people who were of great experience who were nearly broken or on the way to breaking, I don't think they intend to break people or break spirits it is just that it is an occupational hazard in working there [...] it's a breaking from their passion, from their autonomy.

Becoming part of the profession, 'wearing your blues' involved a breaking of one's spirit and a breaking from the philosophy of midwifery as an autonomous profession where midwives have the agency to respond authentically to women's needs.

Autonomy for women and autonomy for student midwives are potentially linked at a conscious and at an unconscious level in a parallel process. The midwife who cannot speak for herself may not encourage women to speak up and the production-line mentality is likely to remain unchallenged. Or indeed, when students think for themselves in a non-encouraging environment they are left potentially exposed to emotional distress. It is likely that the same distress is experienced by women who are non-compliant in robotic care environments.

'No man's land'

The student midwife is in a liminal state between being a layperson and a qualified midwife and, as we have outlined, is caught between competing ideologies which midwives themselves find difficult to manage. Can she be 'with woman', or must she be 'with institution' (Hunter 2004)? Midwife, or '*medwife*' (Cebulak, 2012)? At the same time as managing these tensions, students have the task of learning to be psychologically present for women alongside the elemental emotions evoked by birth. The midwife's role involves becoming a psychological container of powerful feelings for a mother and providing a safe space for her to process her anxieties (Taylor, 2010). When the students experienced continuity and support from clinical mentors within good working relationships, they too experienced support and containment.

Although there were instances of appropriate containment for mothers and students, the powerful empathy felt by student midwives for the women was generally difficult to manage in a busy obstetric unit and increased students' vulnerability:

> *They* [the women] *are the people I feel I can trust to be honest –* [laughs] *but you don't want to get too close because ultimately somebody might come in and do something that will really hurt them and I've got to emotionally back away from that then. So you are kind of in a bit of a no man's land with that, it's strange really.*

When women suffered unnecessarily, student midwives felt that they had betrayed them and blamed themselves for this:

> *I just thought if she spoke English none of that, it probably could have happened to her but she wouldn't have been treated the way that she was treated and I … I … felt really bad that it happened and I do* [tearfully] *blame myself for not stopping it really.*

This 'moral distress' as defined by Jameton (1984) comprises negative feelings that arise when one knows the ethically appropriate response but feels unable to carry it out due to institutional constraints. There is a difference between distress and moral distress – for example, a student could be emotionally distressed from witnessing a traumatic birth but feel morally distressed if the trauma was caused by or exacerbated by health professionals (for example, through disrespectful treatment), and the student felt unable to advocate for the woman. The moral distress and its impact on the students were evident in the study. Some students described their fear of speaking out for themselves and what they believed to be right:

> *It does mean that you are powerless even though you know and you have been told, read, that evidence is, that you should treat certain conditions with certain behaviours this way, or women labour better standing up, these sorts of things. Even if you say that, even if you can convince a midwife to do that sort of thing she can pull the rug straight out from underneath you … can be easily dismissed.*

> *… and it's quite hard to witness that on a daily basis and not feel you can do very much.*

I think, seeing people in situations that I can't do anything for them almost that … that's when you can't control things, or if the people you are working with may not do things to help, and where you feel powerless … that's very difficult.

Students in this study were working long hours, often without breaks, in situations where they had little control over events. Feeling powerless, allied to the close relationships they formed with women may have amplified their vulnerability. Often a distressing episode may have taken place with a woman with whom the student strongly identified, perhaps one of the women she was following through pregnancy, birth and postnatally as part of her own continuity caseload (NMC, 2009). In these situations students described feeling voiceless and complicit in the betrayal of women but had no opportunity to address this moral distress in their training.

Emergency and unforeseen situations

The intense empathy students felt for women rendered them particularly vulnerable in emergency situations. In the quote below, the student included herself in the familial 'we':

And they were both crying, and I said "Can I hug you?" And she said "Oh please, yeah please, will you hug me?" and I gave the dad a hug and I was just like "I don't know what happened, but I'm just so sorry". And they [the parents] *said, "Well we've not got a name for a little…" and I was like, "Right ok, so we've got to have a name, can't leave without a name…"*

The students who had faced clinical emergencies they had found traumatic described long periods of doubt and worry about their role in these emergencies.

I was … wanting answers to why it happened you know, because she had no risk factors for it, so I didn't quite understand why it happened and I think it changed my practice a bit because I was wary; everyone I had I was wary, is something going to go wrong? and it kind of made me withdraw from what I love doing. It took quite a while to get back to normal and just accept that.

Witnessing trauma affected students' confidence to perform their day-to-day duties. For some there was an abiding fear of revisiting places or activities that recalled the event:

Still terrified of being in a labour room on my own really. I know like when we talk about one-to-one midwifery my initial reaction is absolutely not … I do think this has impacted on how I felt because before that I was … they could stand at the door you know leave us alone it's normal … and from that it was actually, I quite like that emergency buzzer there.

When they encountered traumatic events, there was little time or no safe space in the institution in which to reflect and learn from them. Formal support for the students' emotional well-being in practice was rarely depicted as adequate. Similarly to the midwives discussed in Sally Pezaro and colleagues' (2016) exploration of midwives' traumatic experiences, midwives appeared to carry on and soak up difficult events without access to others. A culture of silence was the norm and this heightened participants' self-blame and sense of being emotionally inadequate. Self-blame was exacerbated in a blame culture:

> it was all about, blame......) it turned from being traumatic to this real resounding emotion of fear – it was tangible – you know, who's done it, whose fault is it, who's to blame, ... who's to blame? And that, that also put me off midwifery a lot, cos where I felt like it's a caring profession we'd rally round, it was then more finger-pointing...

Students are likely to be vulnerable as they go through the journey of socialisation into a profession dealing with life and death (Werner and Korsch 1976). The student midwives in our study were rendered particularly vulnerable because of the passionate empathy they felt with the women in their care, reinforced professionally but played out within an institutional framework that largely denied the possibility of authentic caring relationships. They felt hurt when women were hurt and they also spoke of blaming themselves when things went wrong, feeling that they should have been able to protect the women.

The absence of protection and support for students in their navigation of the role pointed up a lack of professional containment. The students in the study often did not feel accepted or valued for the role they played. The outlets available for them to talk through events were patchy. The cultural message perceived by these students was to soldier on or be labelled as problematic or inadequate.

Anxieties in practice

The defences against distress in the profession may, in part, be generated by the closeness the midwives experience with women in their care. Student midwives, anxious in their work environments, may be prone to unconsciously splitting off their concerns; championing women over colleagues; and seeing the environment in black and white terms. This splitting may play into the valid sense of alienation they carried about the job. To learn to tolerate the different emotional pulls within the psychologically fierce environment of labour requires a language with which to situate the distress; this language needs to be socially, politically and psychologically astute. The anxieties in practice internalised negatively by the student relate both to the environment of care and to their individual experiences within the role.

The truths of working as a midwife must include an acknowledgement of loss and limitation to the role as well as to the vicissitudes of the birth process. To be able to name the perils of under-identification with women leading to emotional shutdown and coldness may help student midwives to understand their colleagues. To be alert to the dangers of over-identification leading to a failure to retain openness to a variety of outcomes to the labour process may be important facets of their learning. Also, an ability to consider their potential vulnerability to over-identification and strategies to manage it may enable them to think creatively about their boundaries and the balance they need to strike in order to honour their vision.

Conclusions

The attempt to provide relational care in an organisation geared towards a business-style mode of management results in damaging tensions for students, midwives and mothers. Student midwives have particular vulnerabilities on their journeys to being qualified midwives due to the intense empathy and identification they feel with women, coupled with their relative powerlessness as learners. The traumatic events they recounted took place within a litigious and blaming culture where there were staff shortages and a lack of time or place for midwives and students to make sense of these events together. To address the distress this causes, midwifery needs to develop the psychological language to help students give voice to their individual experiences, to explore the complexities of the midwifery role, and to develop appropriate coping strategies. It also requires political analysis of the wider impact of neoliberalism on the individual, on public services and on midwifery. Both are essential if the student midwife is to successfully traverse the hazardous 'no man's land' of initial midwifery education.

7

THE TRAUMA WOMEN EXPERIENCE AS THE RESULT OF OUR CURRENT MATERNITY SERVICES

Nadine Edwards

Based on women's birth stories, this chapter discusses why women's voices are often muted within maternity services. It shows that this can have traumatic consequences for women's physical and emotional well-being and can undermine their confidence as new parents. For some women, this results in long-term health problems which impact detrimentally on them and on their relationships with family and others (Reed *et al.*, 2017). It suggests why midwives are unable to overcome the impact of an institutionalised, medicalised and fragmented system of maternity care (with stunning exceptions) and give the care they want to give, and what needs to change.

Of course, women recognise and appreciate the efforts made by midwives to give them the best care they can while they are unsupported themselves (www.independent.co.uk/news/uk/home-news/nhs-midwife-open-letter-i-wish-i-was-dead-stress-on-staff-a7375391.html). Since March 2017, this has worsened, with the withdrawal of midwifery supervision which (at its best) was able to support midwives to provide individualised care to women, even when they made decisions outside usual policies and practices. Midwives and women are more constrained than ever by faceless and often hidden bureaucratic, technocratic and obstetric ideologies and structures that reduce women's and midwives' agency; discount the value of relationships and caring (Kirkham, 2017a; Mander and Murphy-Lawless, 2013); and even fall down on their own (limited) criteria of evidence-based care (Prusova *et al.*, 2014).

About the Pregnancy and Parents Centre

The two stories below come from women who attended pregnancy groups at the Pregnancy and Parents Centre, a local charity in central Edinburgh which offers support to over 500 pregnant women and families each week (including a high percentage for whom English is a second language). It is described in more detail in Chapter 11 of this book. One of the aims of the Centre is to increase women's confidence in their abilities to give birth and become capable mothers, and to support new parents. Women attending the pregnancy groups often comment that they feel less afraid of birth and more confident about coping in labour. But with no continuity of midwifery carer, many go into an obstetric unit in labour and are unable to put what they planned into practice. The fragmented, busy system has little time or scope to listen to or support them to birth their babies in their own time and in their own ways, especially if labour does not follow a prescribed trajectory. In other words, the system has little ability to listen to their knowledge or agency, which can result in emotional and physical trauma despite the fact that the National Confidential Enquiries have repeatedly urged practitioners to listen to women.

Women's stories from the Pregnancy and Parents Centre are diverse but the scenarios here are not uncommon and both highlight what can happen when services are overly standardised and busy and when women and midwives have not been able to build trusting relationships. Institutionalised care focused on 'through-put', guidelines, policies and protocols undermines caring and individual voices.

Scenarios

Woman 1 was expecting her third baby, having had two previous quick births of three hours and one-and-a-half hours. She anticipated another fast birth. Through-out pregnancy she 'didn't have a single appointment with the same person'. At term her waters broke, she went to hospital and was allocated a room in the alongside Birth Centre. She went for a few walks and told the midwives that she was having a 'lot of contractions' and that the baby was coming quite soon. The midwives didn't agree and wanted her to go home and come back later for an induction of labour because her waters had broken. She replied that 'to me this baby is about to come out' and she wanted to stay on the premises. She was allowed to stay in the room. The shift changed and the woman reiterated that she felt that her baby was going to be born quite soon. The new midwife said that in her experience third babies do not follow the pattern of previous births and that she should prepare herself for a long labour. The woman acknowledged the midwife's experience but said she felt the baby was coming quite soon. She was using a hypnobirthing tape and pacing in circles because she found this helpful. The midwife questioned this, and 'stood in the way so that I had to go round her' and asked 'What's this hypno-birthing all about?' She then 'grabbed' the woman's abdomen to feel a contraction and said 'Was that it? That wasn't a strong one'. The woman replied, 'It was', to which the midwife said it did not feel like it to her and that it felt as if she was 'nowhere close to labour'. The woman was confused, as she felt close to giving birth. The midwife then decided that as the labour was not progressing she would have to move to the maternity unit and wait for an induction. The woman agreed, assuming that she would be allocated a different midwife in the labour ward as she knew her baby would come soon. She was having 'big' contractions on the way to the ward but was shocked to find herself in a 'shared ward with four families and lots of people around'. She asked where the labour room was, as she was about to give birth, and she was told that someone would be right with her. She repeatedly rang the buzzer but no one came. Finally, a midwife did come and the woman explained that she needed a private room, as she was about to give birth and did not want to birth 'in front of all these people'. The midwife said that the previous midwife had explained the situation to her, that she was due to be induced, that she would be examined in a few hours, to wait patiently, and that there were no rooms anyway. The woman asked to go back to the Birth Centre but was told she must wait until she was induced. The midwife said she would come back, but did not. The woman gave birth a short time later. She was standing by the bed, squatted down and cried out as the baby's head came out. Her husband was pressing the buzzer and shouting 'is no one going to help my wife, she's about to give birth, come and help us', but no one responded until a cleaning woman came by and she went to get the midwife. The midwife asked what the 'drama' was and the woman said the baby's head was out. The midwife said, 'well, let's examine you shall we – hop up on the bed' and was shocked to find the baby's head was out and that the woman had known exactly what was happening in her labour. She said, 'Oh you're much further along than I thought'. So the midwife and the woman's husband ran with the bed 'like mad' down the busy corridor with 'a sea of people' looking at her 'roaring' as she gave birth. Once they arrived in a room, she was told 'well done that lady – they didn't even know my name'. Nor did anyone know where her notes were. She said that she and her baby were healthy, but 'as an experience it was not good'. She was 'over the moon' with her baby, but 'was really angry about how I'd been treated and not been listened to'. The woman felt that her traumatic experience would have been avoided had she been listened to and able to remain in the Birth Centre. She wrote a letter of complaint and received an apology.

Woman 2 had a first healthy pregnancy and felt excited and confident about giving birth (her own mother had seven babies naturally). Short contractions started just after 39 weeks, her waters broke and contractions became stronger, longer and closer together. She phoned the hospital and was asked to phone back when the contractions were closer together. When they were five minutes apart she phoned and was asked to come in. She felt very positive and was looking forward to meeting her baby. The midwife she saw was a 'disappointment' as she was not welcoming and wanted her to take a paracetamol or other drugs, which she had wanted to avoid – 'so that put me down'. She was examined and told that she was not in labour and had to go home. She felt she was not being listened to or responded to and while she had felt:

> very strong and very positive until that moment [...] suddenly I wasn't sure about anything anymore, I was just in big pain and when she said that I wasn't in labour I didn't know what to think or what to do ... so we went back home.

By three in the morning she was in 'unbearable' pain and went back to the hospital. She had another vaginal examination from the same midwife and was told that her cervix had not dilated. She did not want to go home, as she was in extreme pain, felt stressed and did not want to be alone, so she asked if there was a room she could use. She was told she could stay in the parking area, and that she would be induced later, and to take pain killers. She started to cry, as she had hoped things would unfold naturally. She also knew that paracetamol would not relieve the pain but would slow things down. The midwife said it did not matter because she was going to be induced later anyway. She went home and took the paracetamol and another pain killer she had been given. This did not help. Her induction was planned for the evening and she felt happier, as she knew the midwife would no longer be on shift. When she went back everyone was friendly and understood her concerns and explained that she was in so much pain because her baby was back to back, and that because her pregnancy was so healthy she might still be able to use the Birth Centre and have a natural birth. She was seen after an hour and told that she could not use the Birth Centre but could still try for a natural birth, but 'I didn't feel like that anymore because I had to be monitored and I couldn't move, I couldn't stand, I had to be in bed and it was unbearable'. She decided to have diamorphine which helped for a while but her cervix was just one centimetre open. The midwife said she had to be induced and the woman decided to have the epidural she had hoped to avoid. She was able to control the epidural so that she could feel contractions and was able to push and give birth to her son. She and her baby were physically well, but 'I was still very upset a few months later'. She could not stop thinking about the birth and 'felt very sad and disappointed'. Breastfeeding was difficult because her baby had a tongue-tie. This was not recognised at first and she had conflicting advice from different people. So despite feeling strong before the birth about what she wanted to do, 'I felt very insecure and I really felt I didn't know what to do any more'. Reflecting months later, she felt that things might well have gone differently had she been treated differently the first time she went to hospital in labour. Her husband sent a letter of complaint and was informed that there would be an investigation but was later told that the investigation found nothing amiss with what happened.

Women's experiences of birthing are etched into their bodies and minds and have long-term consequences. In Penny Simkin's (1991) research on long-term memories of birth, 'Women reported that their memories were vivid and deeply felt. Those with highest long-term satisfaction ratings thought that they accomplished something important, that they were in control, and that the birth experience contributed to their self-confidence and self-esteem'. Conversely, negative experiences could result in post-traumatic stress disorder, depression, relationship difficulties, avoidance of future pregnancies, and future elective caesarean sections (Lundgren et al., 2009; Nieuwenhuijze et al., 2013).

Contextualising the scenarios: Why does this happen?

The 'irresistibility' of medicalisation

We know that the best care is provided by skilled midwives managing their own caseload with easy access to good obstetric and other services. The evidence for this is overwhelming and accumulating by the day. It is now policy across the UK (NHS England, 2016; Scottish Government, 2017), but remains to be implemented. Meanwhile, as the Scottish Maternity Review notes: 'Normal births have declined steadily, and there has been a rise in interventions, largely from a rise in caesarean sections to 31.1% of all births in 2015' (Scottish Government, 2017).

The reasons for this are complex but one aspect of the ideologies and structures surrounding birth is how they demand conformity from doctors, midwives and women alike (as other chapters in this book demonstrate). When Mandie Scamell (Machin and Scamell, 1997) carried out her research twenty years ago, she concluded that the medicalised approach to birth is 'irresistible' – no matter what the woman's plans before birth. This is consistently confirmed by women's reports over the last two decades:

> If you're in hospital and sometime in the past you've thought, this is what I'd really like to do, it just goes completely out of the window once you're actually in hospital being told what to do by staff, because they think it's best' (Edwards, 2005: 228).

It is borne out by birth stories (Quashie, 2015), *AIMS* articles (www.aims.org.uk) and surveys (Birthrights, 2013). It is extraordinarily difficult for women to make their voices heard above the protocols, policies, institutionalised routines of day-to-day practice, and busyness because the services are unable to make space for them, even when they have serious concerns (Mackintosh *et al.*, 2015; Rance *et al.*, 2013).

Midwives can find it equally difficult to provide good care and voice their concerns (Edwards *et al.*, 2016) and often suffer themselves from trauma and distress (Coldridge and Davies, 2017; Leinweber *et al.*, 2017a) as chapters in this book demonstrate. Doctors also find it increasingly difficult (www.bbc.co.uk/programmes/b08crzrc).

Most practitioners do their utmost to compensate for a flawed maternity system that systematically increases interventions, costs and emotional harms and distress to women and midwives. Intersecting strands (for example, staff and resource shortages, centralisation, standardisation) that flow from contemporary neoliberal ideological and organisational structures reinforce a technocratic approach, the growth of which has been well-documented for three-and-a-half decades. This approach leaves no space for genuinely caring relationships: the hallmark of good midwifery that opens spaces for women to birth in their own time and way (Mander and Murphy-Lawless, 2013). The current system strongly militates against women being listened to, having any agency and avoiding interventions. It cannot improve outcomes and it compromises safety, as demonstrated in the stories above. How can midwives give consistently good care when they are beset by the pressures of understaffing, bullying cultures, guidelines that act as rules, high rates of epidurals, little agency, and when they do not know the women or their aspirations (Kirkham, 2007; 2017b).

The human consequences of these spiralling harms to women and midwives are a travesty. Women are processed and left to get on with their lives as best they can (Kitzinger, 2006) and midwives leave due to stress (Hughes, 2017) or adapt in negative ways by disengaging from those they started off wanting to care for (Deery and Kirkham, 2007).

What improves women's experiences?

Challenging work by feminists and birth activists since the late 1970s has consistently defined the potential of women to be strong givers of birth. By contrast, much conventional academic and service-based policy and evaluation research that reinforces existing social and institutional hierarchies (with women at the bottom), omits to ask women about their thoughts and experiences. Increasingly, mainstream researchers have come to understand that even when defining women in the most limited ways possible as 'recipients' or 'consumers' of care rather than agents of their own labours and births, women are *still* well-placed to comment on our maternity services and how these impact on them.

Women coming to the Pregnancy and Parents Centre want and value the support of their midwives. They want to see the same midwife during their pregnancies, births, and postnatally so they can share and explore their individual circumstances, concerns and aspirations. Some are shocked to learn in early pregnancy that this is not how maternity services are organised.

When women get to know and trust a midwife who provides care throughout their childbearing journey, physical and emotional safety for mothers and babies is more likely to be achieved (Homer *et al.*, 2017; Sandall, Coxon *et al.*, 2016); costs to the NHS are reduced (Schroeder *et al.*, 2012); and women's and midwives' agency is enhanced (McCourt and Stevens, 2009). For women, this is because most find it easier to exert agency in collaboration with supportive others. 'Having an influence together with others, such as their midwife or their partners, was related to a higher sense of control than having an influence only by themselves' (Nieuwenhuijze *et al.*, 2013). In the context of trusting relationships, women describe very positive experiences, even when birth does not unfold straightforwardly (Reed, 2016). Interestingly, a small study suggested that case loading by midwives who support each other can improve women's experiences of birth, even in an obstetric unit (Carolan-Olah *et al.*, 2015).

Had the two women above been able to build mutually trusting relationships with their midwives, they would have been listened to and believed. The first woman would have had the same joyful and straightforward birth with her third baby as she had had with her previous two babies. The second woman may have been able to avoid interventions, but had these become necessary she would have felt cared for and content that all had been done to support her, rather than distressed and sad about her baby's birth. Both would have emerged strong, confident and ready to meet the challenges of new motherhood without having to deal with distressing emotions and lengthy complaints.

We have an opportunity across the UK to move towards services that women want and which have been shown beyond doubt to improve outcomes, their experiences, and those of midwives. The policy documents produced across the UK support the introduction of continuity of carer, as did the policy review in England and Wales in 1992 (House of Commons, 1992) but there were insufficient resources and a lack of political will to mainstream and sustain this.

Midwifery, good birth, and women's experiences hang in the balance: we now know a great deal more than we did in the 1990s about the benefits of case loading midwifery care. Making the community and relationship with a midwife, who is herself supported, the bedrock of maternity services cannot be left to the machinations of bureaucracy but needs to be acted on without delay. We cannot afford to let families down again but it will take political will, adequate resources, training, support, listening to women, and most of all a groundswell of opinion and activism to move towards a community-based accessible and equitable maternity service that genuinely cares for all families irrespective of their circumstances.

8
WHEN MIDWIVES BECOME OTHER

Helen Shallow

Background

As a head of midwifery and consultant midwife, I was concerned by the increasing regularity with which mothers who chose to birth in hospital reported that they had not been listened to and were not believed when they knew their labours had begun. Some mothers were repeatedly turned away and told that they were not in labour because their cervix (neck of the womb), had not opened more than four centimetres (NICE, 2014: 17). Being turned away, often in significant pain, caused some mothers substantial fear and distress. Other mothers arrived in advanced labour after being told to stay at home, and some mothers birthed unexpectedly either at home or en route to hospital, causing them deep distress and post-traumatic stress (Greenfield *et al.*, 2016). All these mothers were denied the support and pain relief that they had been assured of throughout pregnancy, presenting both a safety and a quality issue. I sought to understand what prevented midwives offering the support to mothers that was evidently needed and expected.

The mothers' narratives reflect concerns raised in other parts of this book. This chapter focuses on midwives' experiences, as their experiences are less-well documented when they are implicated in mothers' unhappy births. Their accounts highlight the potential for long-term psychological damage, working as they do within a maternity service in crisis.

Context

The rhetoric of successive government documents represents the NHS as a, 'modern', 'dependable' and 'liberated' public service (DoH, 2012, 2010, 1997). Yet successive governments, NHS managers and bureaucrats prioritise cost efficiency over quality of care as they deliver on a neoliberal policy to privatise health care (Pollock and Price, 2011; Pollock, 2005).

Oxymoronic pairings such as 'cost effectiveness and quality improvement', deliberately promoted by certain elements of the media, are designed to make us believe that health and social care has never been better when in reality the NHS is being dismantled (Mander and Murphy-Lawless, 2013: 121). As a result, midwives have become gatekeepers to a restricted service and are reluctant to involve mothers in decision-making for fear of being overwhelmed. As their accounts demonstrate, they are caught between mothers' expressed needs and organisational demands to increase throughput and to vacate beds.

Study details

The 'Are you listening to me?' study took place in a district general hospital in the north of England between 2012 and 2015 (Shallow, 2016). Maternity services comprised one obstetric unit, a co-located birth centre and a freestanding birth centre. The annual birth rate was just over 6,000. Seventy-two mothers and midwives took part in the study. My choice of methodology, participatory action research (Brydon-Miller *et al.*, 2011), was born out of a feminist endeavour to give voice to mothers and midwives, and to raise awareness, as well as affording midwives a safe space to share their perspectives. After a series of interviews and focus groups, midwives were invited to a joint one-day workshop with mothers to discuss preliminary findings and make recommendations

Midwives becoming other

The focus of my study was the interactions between mothers and midwives when labour begins. This chapter examines midwives' experiences as they grappled with the realities of daily practice.

No time: Interactions as distractions

Mothers in early labour generally phone the obstetric unit or the birth centre. Midwives have no dedicated time to talk to these mothers, so telephone and face-to-face interactions and admission assessments are carried out in and among other activities of the labour ward/triage or birth centre/midwife-led setting. Midwives know that being positive, introducing themselves, listening to and giving the mother time, improve mothers' experiences, but they have no time:

> It's having the time to listen and the time to focus in.

This midwife went on to describe how she would have to 'zone out' all the extraneous noise and ongoing activity in order to be able to stop and listen, and focus on what the mother was telling her. Having no time was a particular feature on the labour ward, described as a 'conveyor belt':

> You don't get that luxury [of time] on labour ward. It's like a conveyor belt of mothers.

Another midwife commented:

> Usually if you're in triage you're already admitting someone or half way through looking after that mother when the phone's ringing and you're having to excuse yourself from that job when you're halfway through, to answer the phone and you feel very conscious about the person you've left behind who's you know, who's distressed or...

A midwife added that taking a phone call meant abruptly leaving a mother and subsequently:

> somebody's maybe waiting for a speculum [examination] under a sheet [...] behind crappy curtains'.

Midwives talked mostly of the 'distraction' of telephone interactions, because these 'distractions' led to disjointed and unfocused care for mothers already being cared for, as well as for those at the end of the phone. Despite knowing that they needed time to interact with mothers meaningfully, their accounts described functioning in a production-line system, where mothers and their needs in early labour have little place and become an unwanted distraction from the processing of women through the system as quickly as possible. The hospital management system 'visual hospital' (www.visualhospital.co.uk) introduced to 'improve hospital flow' has added pressure on midwives to keep mothers out of hospital or send them home if they are not considered to be in active labour, that is, the woman's cervix is not four centimetres dilated.

Distracted focus

Midwives depicted the complex emotional 'switching and swapping faces' reported on by Deery (2010). They described the difficulty they had switching their focus from one interactive activity to another. A midwife portrayed this 'emotional labour' as:

> switching yourself off from what you've just been doing there to starting afresh with whoever is on the phone and whatever they're ringing with.

One midwife talked about how she tries to focus by blocking out the activity around her:

> And when that phone rings in triage and you're really busy, not that I mind taking the phone call but my heart sinks. I think, "I don't have time for this". It's like a bit

of a desperation and I've had to learn to make sure the rest of the mothers are okay, go to the phone and block out everything that's going on and to give that mother, you know some nice, calm, a length of time, advice and help because you literally have to block out everything that's going on. Obviously sometimes you can't because you might get a deceleration and you have to tell that mother "just bear with me, I'll be back in a second, I just have to go check on…" but it is, it's really stressful.

Others found this difficult as they had no 'thinking time':

also I just find thinking time, you know if your head is so full how can you really [do] what you want to do on the phone because you're in so short time, you want to make a quick decision and sometimes it's not that quick decision.

She compared this to a good interaction where:

It's about counselling on the phone and erm, so then you don't do the counselling, you do the quick decision which is more for your benefit at that moment, not the benefit of the mother.

In other words, due to workload pressures, the midwife, albeit unintentionally, was meeting her own need to cope, rather than interacting in a meaningful way with the mother at the other end of the line. It is little wonder that some mothers experienced phone calls and face-to-face interactions as perfunctory, and reported that they were not being listened to.

While most midwives maintained that it was better for mothers to go home or stay at home in early labour, some believed this should be the mother's decision and that, despite seeking advice, it was the mother who best understood her needs and whether or not to go home. This is a key factor in mothers' perceptions of maintaining control and feeling satisfied with their care (Carlsson *et al.*, 2012; Fahy, 2002). However, it appeared that midwives had very little control over the work environment or the decisions they or mothers might or might not make.

Working in the worst place

Many first interactions with mothers in early labour occur in triage. Midwives reported that this was the worst place to work, especially during busy times. Introduced to maternity from emergency services in the early millennium, triage originates from the task of assessing the most injured on the battlefield. In maternity triage, a mother may present and wait her turn, sometimes for hours before she is seen. Only if her birth is imminent will she be able to jump the queue. Maternity triage has become a gate-keeping service to the labour ward. Admission may only be achieved by fulfilling prescribed parameters. The most significant of which is dilatation of the cervix.

A midwife summed up the general view:

Triage? I hate it. At best it is tolerable, at worst it's deplorable.

...and the pressure to multi-task

As a senior midwife responsible for staff allocation, one midwife commented that an 'experienced' midwife who could 'multi-task' and use a measure of 'common sense', as well as being 'personable' would be able to manage the work in triage. However, 'managing' the workload in triage meant suppressing midwives' values and beliefs, causing anxiety and distress to many midwives in this study.

Donning an impenetrable suit of armour

During a focus group a midwife stood up to demonstrate the 'midwife's walk' on a standard shift on labour ward and triage. With double-quick steps, she bowed her shoulders, lowered her head and marched forward. It was as if she had donned a heavy suit of armour. In this one action she illustrated how impenetrable her body language was to a mother seeking support. Several midwives added that they avoided eye contact:

I don't like how it changes how you are sometimes. You know sometimes if you've got a lot of people on the corridor waiting, you've got all your beds full, you don't want to make eye contact with anybody.

Another midwife made reference to the pressure midwives are under, especially pertaining to burgeoning paperwork and clinical governance where 'the collective control of work based on guidelines and protocols' prevails (Scamell and Stewart, 2014: 84):

an enormous amount of midwifery now is about self-protection and not about being a good midwife.

Formulaic responses as self-protection

In order to cope with impossible workloads, midwives needed mothers to remain at home irrespective of their wishes and, according to the mothers, gave standardised, bland, formulaic responses when they phoned up in labour. Even if they were concerned, anxious, fearful, or in pain, they were often told:

that's normal, you're fine, have a paracetamol and a bath.

Or,

well you can come in but if you're not as far on as ... you'll have to go.

Midwives used these responses to avoid further engagement when their workloads were demanding and they occasionally missed situations that were not 'normal'. In addition, recommending staying at home and taking medication not only has the potential to inhibit labour progress (Hughes, 2015), it fails to utilise the therapeutic effect their own presence could have on reducing mothers' fear, anxiety and pain (Edwards, 2005).

The need to conform

While standard responses were experienced negatively by mothers, midwives felt the 'irresistible' pressure of a socialisation process (Hunt and Symonds, 1995) that demands conformity:

> *Okay, well, when you work on labour ward which is kind of where I did my basic training, if you like, post registration training, it's very difficult not to get into that sort of,* [said with ironic staccato tone of voice] *"midwife labour ward" voice … I think that you do it automatically, because you want to fit in with the rest.*

Another midwife commented that:

> *even if you're looking at people and thinking "I don't want to sound like that on the phone, I don't want to be that midwife" you know you almost do assume that role because you're surrounded by that.*

One midwife described the difficulty of practising midwifery differently, even in the birth centre where midwives might spend time with mothers in early labour and offer them a lavender bath to help them relax. However:

> *I would feel a bit silly going up to the co-ordinator* [on labour ward] *and saying "oh I've got this lady in triage who I don't want to assess yet, she's just you know come in and she's maybe wanting to have a bath" and then I honestly I'd be looked at like "are you actually joking?"*

In effect, the midwife felt she had to alter how she practised, depending on whether she was working in a birth centre within a social model or on labour ward within an industrial model, focused on throughput.

One-to-one, or one-to-everyone, or one-to-no one?

The intrapartum care guideline for well women in labour recommends one-to-one care for mothers in 'active labour' (NICE, 2014). It became evident from the data that midwives interpreted one-to-one care differently, depending on their workload and where they worked.

Some midwives developed a pragmatic approach to one-to-one care as another form of self-protection and might only spend time with a mother for as long as it took to take and record clinical observations, such as blood pressure, pulse, fetal heart pattern and number of contractions:

> *I can dip in and out and do the care, do the obs, you don't have to stay* [with a mother].

One midwife described the good team player as the midwife who could multi-task, help her colleagues and 'skip about', providing some care to all, rather than all care to one. She emphasised that at least all mothers received some care – though for mothers this kind of approach resulted in inappropriate or inadequate support.

Other midwives talked about the conflicting responsibilities and challenges they faced. In the birth centres there may be two midwives on duty and two mothers in 'active' labour requiring one-to-one support. If another mother called seeking admission, one midwife discussed what observations she might expect to make and document and what care she would be expected to provide and document. If the mother was admitted, and she could not physically be with her while providing one-to-one care for the other mother in labour, she would be failing in her duty of care. She conceded that in circumstances where she considered the mother to be 'not in labour' it was safer for her to delay admission. After all, she commented:

> *It's my registration and if I let her in, I have to be responsible.*

There was a perception that if the mother did not cross the hospital threshold the midwife could not be held responsible.

Working against beliefs and values

Midwives do not come into midwifery to compromise their practice or give poor care, and yet they described the compromises necessary to survive the daily workload. Delivering good care was at times impossible as they 'skipped about' and 'dipped in and out' wearing a suit of armour that disconnected them from mothers, in response to the pressures around them.

One midwife talked about her experience when a senior labour ward midwife tried to coerce her to examine a mother with a view to sending her home:

> *I think as well … it's going back, but it's kind of erm, the conversation as well. "Have you VE'd her?" when we're talking about latent phase mothers "well no I don't need to VE her just yet", we're talking, we're chatting and then you know we might have another phone call and "what's that mother doing, have you VE'd her yet?", "no we're talking about what's happening to her body".*

And a lead midwife described how she found herself in an impossible position:

> *It's frustrating … and at times it's frightening. There's been times when you are down to the last bed on labour ward and I mean this is absolutely horrendous, down to the last bed on labour ward and going and waking mothers up at 3.00 in the morning asking if they'd like to go home because that's what you've been told to do by the managers further up.*

When asked how it felt to work against their values and beliefs, two midwives exchanged these views:

> Midwife 1. *Crap, … I don't want to work like that. I don't want to work like that on a regular basis. You know there will be days where it happens, that happens on the birth centres as well.*

> Midwife 2. *What does that do to you?*

> Midwife 1. *The crap makes me feel like I'm a bad midwife; a bad person and I don't want to do it.*

> Midwife 2. [It] *damages you as a person.*

And another midwife commented:

> *yeah there's no job satisfaction at all. You don't feel like you're caring for anybody, you're not doing your role for anyone and you just feel like you're walking around apologising and feeling guilty all the time that you're not providing the care you want to give because you can't, you're spread too thinly.*

I examined the psychological impact of midwives not being able to work as they wanted and trying to reconcile the irreconcilable through the theory of cognitive dissonance (Cooper, 2007).

Cognitive dissonance theory

Cognition refers to the mental process by which external or internal input is 'transformed, reduced, elaborated, stored, recovered and used' (Brandimonte, Bruno and Collina, 2006: 14). So cognitive dissonance results when: 'a feeling of discomfort leads to an alteration in one of the [previously held] attitudes, beliefs or behaviours [in order to] reduce the discomfort and restore balance' (McLeod, 2014: 1).

For example, irrespective of the mothers' requests for help or support, when 'they are no longer comfortable to stay at home' (Wickham, 2015), midwives in this study continued to tell mothers that staying at home, (without midwifery support), was in their best interests because to tell them otherwise meant they would have to acknowledge their lack of capacity.

Cognitive dissonance theory led to a deeper understanding of the implications of a fractured midwifery service where mothers' needs are not being met and where midwives cannot be the midwives they strive to be, irrespective of where they worked. Some midwives altered their behaviours in order to comply and fit in with the prevailing dominant model most commonly seen on contemporary labour wards. These midwives adopted pragmatic and self-protective measures to get through the work and survive the shift. However, on reflection they realised they were not being the midwives they originally aspired to be. They had become 'other' and even their protective coats of armour were wearing thin. Other midwives, accused of lacking 'resilience', are experiencing severe cognitive dissonance as they struggle to uphold their midwifery values and beliefs in an increasingly toxic environment (Kirkham, 2017b).

Findings from this study indicate that in both the social and technocratic models of midwifery there are barriers to providing safe, satisfactory care that leads to emotional as well as physical well-being, because midwives and mothers are situated within inappropriate, neoliberal organisational structures (Mander and Murphy-Lawless, 2013).

Conclusion

This chapter focused on midwives' interactions with women when labour begins. The data revealed deep and long-lasting harms to midwives as they struggled to be the midwives they aspired to be. It revealed the frictions and fractures in UK maternity care where midwives, irrespective of the model of care or setting, have to adapt, comply or leave, and at the same time experience varying degrees of cognitive dissonance that leave them in a permanent state of conflict or discomfort, knowing as they do that they cannot always provide safe care and best outcomes (Renfrew et al., 2014; Scamell and Stewart, 2014). If the current organisation of maternity services in the UK is not rapidly and comprehensively addressed, more midwives and mothers will become hostage to the misfortunes reported from two recent major NHS investigations (Francis, 2010; Kirkup, 2015). The current risk-averse/efficiency-saving/productivity culture makes these incidents more likely to happen as midwives struggle to survive and eventually retire or leave (Curtis et al., 2006).

The midwives in this study highlighted challenges when faced with fragmented service provision. The latest maternity reviews (NHS England, 2016; Scottish Government, 2017) cannot be shoe-horned into existing configurations. The implementation of continuity of carer in the current UK maternity services is untenable unless basic principles of the mother–midwife partnership underpin a radical restructuring of UK maternity services.

9

FUNDAMENTAL CONTRADICTIONS

The business model versus midwifery values

Mavis Kirkham

It seems to me that many of the current problems around birth are due to a fundamental clash of values. Midwifery is rooted in relationships and a tradition of generosity, which research and long experience has shown to have excellent clinical and social outcomes. Most women can birth well if surrounded by people who value them, listen to them and nurture their self-confidence. The NHS is now run on a commercial model: the imperative being to get more for less. In industry this is termed efficiency: maximum productivity for minimum cost. In any other context it is seen as meanness.

Centralisation

Maternity services have been centralised into large hospitals. Applying principles seen as 'sound' in business terms, units have been closed that would have been seen as large ten years ago. Maternity services are no longer local, women are unlikely to know 'their' midwife, and many face alarmingly long journeys in labour just when they should be feeling safe-and secure.

Centralisation produces economies of scale, or more output for less input and in maternity care the main input is staffing. So midwives are part of a large body of staff who can be moved wherever they are needed; the traditional ebb and flow of smaller-scale units is ironed out to a situation where staff permanently feel they are working flat out. This is reputed to be a very efficient way to run a factory-type production line; but we are dealing with people.

There is something deeply inappropriate about placing the personal and intimate experience of birth in a large institution organised on factory principles. It is often said that the important outcome is a live healthy baby, but relationships and experience are fundamental to health and the nature of experiences around birth and breastfeeding have long-term consequences for family health.

So many studies have shown that women feel they are on a conveyor belt, which they see as synonymous with not being treated as a human being. Midwives feel they are regarded as cogs in a machine and not as people. Midwives value relationships with their clients and with colleagues, so that trust can develop; the bigger the unit and the more that staff are moved about, the more relationships are fragmented. So trust does not develop and fear flourishes in its absence.

Alongside the centralisation of clinical services, midwifery education has moved from being based in the clinical setting to being centralised and academicised into universities. Student midwives still spend around half of their time in clinical settings where they have to achieve specific educational objectives (40 normal births, etc.). Where clinical midwives are torn between the needs of the hospital institution and the needs of and for relationships with clients and colleagues, students are torn in several ways. They are university students with assessments to work for and essays to write but they cannot really be part of wider university life because of their clinical commitments and shift-working patterns. Their powerless position as students makes them particularly vulnerable to the many pressures of the clinical institution (Davies and Coldridge, 2015; Coldridge and Davies, 2017). Challenging the practice they witness in the light of their knowledge of research is difficult when they are challenging those who will assess their practice. They are training to be midwives and want to be accepted as colleagues within the clinical setting, but to achieve this they often find the idealism which motivated them to start the course has to be modified, painfully, as it continues. It is unusual for such conflicts to be addressed and analysed as part of the course, though there are outstanding exceptions. There are few people they can turn to who understand their situation and can help them. Many midwifery lecturers are refugees from the stresses of clinical practice and, while many 'link' organisationally with a clinical setting (Collington et al., 2012), few maintain their own clinical practice and experience its present-day stresses and contradictions.

Control and standardisation

If a large organisation is to be run for maximum efficiency, management control is required to monitor and ensure that efficiency. Midwives cannot be trusted to do midwifery or to decide a woman's care in response to her needs, as this might lead to care being given beyond the 'efficient' norm. Thus standardisation is required.

Standardisation requires care to be defined as a series of tasks to be monitored rather than a continuing supportive relationship. If the required tasks are performed then women can logically be neglected between tasks and the midwife's attention given to other women, even when they feel most vulnerable in labour. Defining labour care as a series of standardised tasks makes it possible to give midwives such heavy workloads that they cannot give individualised care, especially as such deviant care is required to be thoroughly, time-consumingly justified. Standardisation is justified as preventing really bad care but it also prevents really good care from being the norm; though many midwives strive to give good care, often at great cost to themselves. This approach is often described as being evidence-based, but research deals with the general, never stating what an individual needs, and much evidence is based on a consensus of those thoroughly versed in cost-saving.

Ironically, a considerable bureaucracy is needed to monitor the efficiency of a large organisation, so costs rise, leading to further cuts to keep costs under control. Such cuts are seldom made to the bureaucracy, which is seen as essential (Weber, 1946; Graeber, 2015).

Education is similarly closely defined in terms of competencies which make students' learning somewhat task-orientated, and the increasing use of simulation further emphasises technical skills over relationships. Learning outcomes and educational input are clearly stated. Learning hours are measured against outcomes, and learning without staff input saves money. Such a tight focus limits the potential of education and the extent to which students are expected to read around subjects or explore them from many angles. Meanwhile, midwife teachers spend increasing time involved with bureaucratic tasks which limit their availability to students.

Fear and rules

As midwifery is increasingly micromanaged, midwives lose the autonomy and flexibility essential to woman-centred care. Policies, procedures and guidelines rapidly fossilise into rules. Midwives lack the time and energy to justify deviance from such rules. As rules proliferate, both the potential for and the fear of getting it wrong increases. The fear thus generated reinforces the pressure to conform.

There is no evidence that rule-governed practice improves clinical outcomes. Rules cannot be made for every eventuality and the habit of conformity undermines midwives' ability to think out the best course of action when they find themselves in a situation for which there are no rules.

There has always been routinised behaviour in midwifery. Many years ago, when I was a pupil midwife, the routine was justified as 'that is how we do it here' or 'Mr X (the consultant) likes his ladies to have...'. The variety of consultants' foibles demonstrated to midwives that things could be done in different ways and probably fostered the creativity with which the routine could be undermined to help particular women. Standardisation has produced a uniformity that takes courage to undermine.

Student midwives are particularly vulnerable in this regard. They find themselves required to follow the rules in practice while writing in their essays the rhetoric of woman-centred, research-based care that they have been taught. Thus they are trained to fluency in a tragic doublespeak of rhetoric and a very different reality. This parallels the chasm between the policy rhetoric of continuity and woman-centred care (e.g. NHS England, 2016; DoH, 1993) and clinical reality.

Staffing

These pressures damage midwives, as individuals and as a workforce. We have plenty of research on this. Lack of occupational autonomy distresses midwives (Sandall 1998). Midwives leave because they cannot give the care they wish to give (RCM 2016b; Ball *et al.*, 2002), which leads to less staff, which puts further pressure on those who remain and this in turn leads others to leave. As this vicious circle produces job vacancies, the opportunity is often taken to reduce posts and thereby save resources. Outside London, I am not sure whether the problem is a shortage of midwives or a shortage of midwifery posts.

With increasing financial pressures, specialist posts are cut back. This removes midwives who have found their niche and built up expertise and a degree of autonomy in a specialist role and moves them back onto the conveyor belt where they are more likely to leave. It also reduces the help available to mothers.

In education there are constant pressures to increase student numbers and to economise on staffing costs. The ratio of student midwives to midwifery teachers was defended with vigilance for many years but this now seems forgotten. Shared learning between the different professions involved in maternity care seems to be a very good idea but often means a few student midwives in a lecture theatre full of student doctors or nurses listening to a lecture written to meet the needs of the majority profession. In their clinical placements, the needs of students of other professions and the pressures upon their clinical mentors also serve to limit the experience gained by student midwives. Like childbearing women, many student midwives have told me how they often feel that all the staff are just too busy to give them their time or attention.

Commodification and technology

Within the business model, services are seen as commodities. This makes child-bearing women into service users, a strangely passive rendering of the ultimate creative act of giving birth. The focus thus moves from the woman and her birth to the service and its providers. Consumer choice may be lauded but women can only choose from the limited options provided by the service.

In recent years, the focus upon the midwife as service provider has enabled management and service users to blame the individual midwife rather than the system for poor outcomes. Midwives now feel the ever present threat of blame as a weighty pressure upon them.

The commercial model is about selling products. The use of technology and pharmaceuticals has proliferated within maternity care. We still use electronic fetal heart monitors (EFMs) in circumstances where research has shown they do not help and may hinder women in labour. Commercial pressures and the value our society places upon technology have created a real fear of not using all the technology available. Yet interventions in childbirth all carry side effects, financial or medical, which exacerbate the spiral of interventions in maternity care. This can have damaging results for individuals and can greatly increase costs, as with increased caesarean rates with EFM (Nelson *et al.*, 2016).

The status which comes with technology may be one reason why midwives have embraced so many additional technical tasks over the years. Thus a cloak of technology is cast over a very basic human service and midwives come to be seen as skilled technicians who are 'checking not listening' (Kirkham *et al.*, 2002) to women. This warps our language and midwives now speak of 'caring' for women who they see only briefly to record clinical observations (Shallow, 2016). We cannot do everything, though we try hard, and basic supportive care fades in significance or moves into the role of the doula or support worker. Thus we neglect what research shows works best.

The financial pressures on the NHS mean that identifiable parts of the service become separate products. Thus, NHS antenatal classes in many places have been cut to the extent that women have to pay for them outside the NHS. 'Special' antenatal classes, such as hypnobirthing, often have to be paid for. NHS midwives cannot give continuing support to childbearing women, so they employ doulas. Breastfeeding support is available, at a price: the price may be monetary or it may be the time of a generous volunteer.

This commodification of what was once seen as midwifery care provides a safe, if commercially vulnerable, haven for a few midwives and other workers. But it discriminates heavily against those women who cannot afford extras. It also prevents integration of services and continuity of carer.

The move from student bursaries to loans is likely to emphasise education as a commodity, as is already the case in many subject areas. This change also defines student midwives as consumers of education rather than as people training to provide a public service. When students become purchasers of education they want value for money and maximum returns for their investment of money and time. In my experience, this often means students want to know precisely what they have to do to get their qualification and see little point in doing much else. This is a logical response to commodification but it does not foster the intellectual curiosity on which the future of our profession depends.

'Consumerism involves the simplification of roles and their associated tasks, and in so doing fundamentally changes the relation of the subject to the group and the institution' (Long, 2008: 156). This redefinition of roles results in the 'potential and actual loss of learning from the experience that is inherent in the richer role' (ibid.) of midwife, mother or student. Some keep the learning but reject the role; I am struck by the number of midwives now working as doulas and mothers choosing to freebirth.

Insurance

Insurance is probably the ultimate example of a product so well-marketed that it appears unethical not to have it. Yet its main beneficiaries are the insurance companies. Once insurance is required for practitioners, the insurers can control clinical practice. In the USA, managed care is packaged and defined by insurers. In this country the conditions of insurance determine who can receive care from independent midwives, thus excluding many women who seek independent midwives because they find themselves damaged by previous NHS care. And, if regulators decide that insurance is insufficient, care can be removed from women as happened here recently (NMC, 2017).

Above all, this system is unjust. If a child needs special care, that care should be available because the child needs it, not for the reason that it can be funded because someone can be blamed. No-fault compensation works in New Zealand. Midwives there do not understand the problems with insurance here because, once liability for the care of a child is removed, the cost of clinical negligence insurance is manageable for them.

Fear of litigation feeds the climate of fear within NHS obstetrics and midwifery. I have often heard midwives refuse requests for care outside the standard package because 'my registration would be on the line'. Conformity and fear thus reinforce each other.

As well as being unjust, insurance is horrendously expensive, accounting for a high proportion of the cost of each NHS birth. How can clinicians provide an economic service if they have to carry this massive financial burden?

Midwifery values

Midwifery is grounded in relationships and works best where midwives have trusting relationships with women and colleagues. To achieve this we need a degree of professional autonomy and continuity in our relationships with clients and colleagues. Present values of fragmentation and management control thwart these relationships. Midwives' professional commitments to their clients simply lead to their exploitation in the context of commercial values. This is shown where so many work extra unpaid hours rather than abandon vulnerable women.

Trapped in this contradiction between their professional values and those of their employers, NHS midwives are torn apart. They continue trying to do the impossible. Their leaders speak the rhetoric of midwifery while clinical midwives work within the reality of a service aiming for maximum efficiency. They see the needs of the clients but their workload is such that they cannot respond to these needs. This is not a healthy way to live. It damages midwives, makes the most rewarding job in the world highly frustrating, and is unacknowledged as a problem.

The academic values which should underpin midwifery education are similarly undermined by economic and bureaucratic pressures. The early midwifery degrees often took four years. Most midwifery degree programmes included an elective placement which many students chose with care, often fundraising if the placement was distant, and writing about their important experiences afterwards. There are now few electives because the curriculum is so crowded and there is discussion as to whether three-year degree programmes can be shortened.

As a relatively new academic subject, midwifery has a short history of research and the development of concepts and ideas. Nurturing intellectual curiosity requires time and that is a resource in short supply. Bureaucracy tends to strangle intellectual curiosity and midwifery moved into universities just as bureaucracy set in there. Midwife teachers became university lecturers because their jobs moved and they endeavoured to fit in, working hard and gaining PhDs because this was expected of them. Few had the luxury of full-time PhD research on a subject of their choice. Academic midwifery careers almost always mean giving up clinical practice, which limits the possibility of cross-fertilisation between clinical and research work.

In university departments where midwives do research, the pressure to get research funding is immense. Bidding for it is highly competitive and does not foster collaboration. There is little money for researching the issues which arise in midwifery practice, yet some excellent research is done on a shoestring and sometimes involves cutting input into education. Despite all these pressures useful research is done; the Birthplace Study is a great example (Brocklehurst *et al.*, 2011) yet so many of its recommendations are not being implemented because the pressures on clinical services prevent its managers looking at the bigger picture.

Perverted commercial values

The current organisation of NHS maternity services has all the drawbacks of a commercial system plus many negative characteristics that would not be tolerated in business. These anachronisms prevent it from seizing the opportunities offered by the fact that, for most women, midwifery care provides excellent outcomes and may well be cheaper than heavily managed hospital care (Schroeder *et al.*, 2017). How can we have a business model so perversely bureaucratic that it misses the potential for such savings?

It is reasonable to argue that the NHS market model is outdated, being rooted in an early-twentieth-century Taylorist, fragmented model of production long since abandoned in industry as inflexible (e.g. Fairtlough, 1994, 2005; Allan *et al.*, 2002). David Boyle (2011) suggests that, rather than tightening up systems even more, real effectiveness can only happen when people are given whole jobs to do, together with the freedom to innovate. This certainly fits with what we know about midwives' relationships with their work and clients (Kirkham *et al.*, 2006). Yet maternity services are fearfully rule-obsessed.

Management experts have long seen it as essential to 'drive out fear, so that everyone may work effectively' (Scherkenbach, 1986: 79) and state that 'the waste due to fear is enormous' (ibid.). Yet fear, blame and bullying run through NHS maternity services and this corrodes the confidence of all concerned.

There is something deeply perverse about the culture within which NHS maternity services operate. Susan Long (2008: 5) addresses this, highlighting how organisations become divided from the humans populating them, the simultaneous acknowledgement and denial of reality and the 'abusive cycles' that result (2008:

15). This fits a service which was originally offered by individuals and has had many different models grafted on to it over time; the market model being the most recent. This results in a service built on a conflict in values and ossified by subsequent bureaucracy.

The perversity of the present system is unsustainable. In nightmare moments I see it as a step on the way to a completely privatised system as in the USA. Yet USA maternity care is not to be envied.

Care and its impact

Midwifery is a public service which can have a long-term impact on families' lives. This is achieved through care: showing how to change a nappy; or modelling for women who have only interacted with adults the ways in which they can relate to a tiny, totally dependent baby; or just providing approval and a safe space for them to get to know their babies. In Meg Taylor's words:

> the midwife metaphorically holds the mother so she can both literally and metaphorically hold her baby. It is obvious that when women are in labour they need a high level of care and attention, but I think a particular quality of attention continues to be required in the postnatal period ... [thus] ... providing this kind of holding.
>
> *(Taylor 2010: 235)*

In providing such holding, the midwife models the generous, loving care which makes its recipient feel safe. This crucial holding is not possible where care is fragmented, where labour care is divided into a series of monitoring tasks and postnatal support is minimised and thereby seen as efficient. Where care is standardised and fragmented, the midwife's attention is on the task in hand, not the individual mother, and the long-term value of the midwife–mother relationship can be lost.

If midwives are to model trusting relationships and provide empathetic care, they need to receive such care themselves and be trusted in their role. This is not experienced by most NHS midwives and may become less likely as we lose the role of Supervisor of Midwives. Student midwives particularly need to receive the care that they will later give, and to work with midwives who model such care.

The future

The values which underpin the organisation and undermine the purpose of the NHS seem to be all-pervading in the Western world. Yet, while control and penny-pinching may work in business (although experts dispute this), a different ethic is required for public services if those who give and receive services are to flourish.

There are other ways of looking at birth and public services: a guardian model for public services was proposed by Jane Jacobs (1992) or simply a decision by society to support generous services around birth as an investment (in commercial terminology) in the future of its citizens. Addressing only short-term, easily measurable outcomes is not a commitment to the next generation.

A society based on commercial values neglects care at its peril. This can be seen in many places (Fraser, 2016; Ehrenreich and Hochschild, 2002) but nowhere is this more important than at the beginning of life. This is especially clear because birth is something that most women can do supremely well if they are trusted and supported and a good start in life has positive outcomes throughout a family's life.

Continuity of midwifery care would be a good starting point for change, since it produces good clinical outcomes and greater satisfaction for all concerned (Sandall, Soltani et al., 2016) as well as being Department of Health policy (DoH, 1993; NHS England, 2016). Ongoing relationships between midwives and mothers and between colleagues move midwives' immediate loyalty in favour of the women in their care (Brodie, 1996). Such loyalty and the potential for alliances between midwives and mothers could be the beginning of great change. This alliance transformed maternity services in New Zealand (Guilliland and Pairman, 2011). Secure in their relationships with childbearing women as individuals and as a political group, midwives would be less fearful. This could lead to the erosion of the organisational constraints which prevent midwives from concentrating on the women in their care. The educational and economic results could be far reaching.

In supporting normal birth, working in primary health and strengthening family ties (ICM, 2005), midwifery provides a sustainable service and can be seen as a 'truly ecological and socially responsible profession' (Davies et al., 2011: 2). Yet so much that midwives are required to do flies in the face of this. We hear midwives being criticised because they lack resilience. I think it is far more useful to see our current dilemmas as manifestations of a fundamental clash of values and the logic which follows from those values, rather than blaming the individuals who suffer these contradictions. Midwives and mothers together could change this.

This chapter has been developed from an article which appeared in *Midwifery Matters* (www.midwifery.org.uk). I would like to thank Anna Fielder and Sarah Davies for their constructive comments on earlier drafts.

PART III

Responding practically and politically to change our troubled maternity structures

Introduction

In Elizabeth Baines' 1983 novel *The Birth Machine*, the protagonist Zelda escapes from hospital with her baby to regain her sanity after a nightmarish technologised labour and caesarean birth. That phrase 'the birth machine' pinpointed what women and midwives were coming to identify as critically wrong with our maternity structures. The World Health Organization (WHO) director of maternal health, Marsden Wagner, writing *Pursuing The Birth Machine* a decade later, scrupulously detailed these damaging consequences alongside the failures of entrenched medical, scientific and public policy establishments – nationally, internationally, and locally – to respond adequately: 'The problem is that the birth machine is out of control' (Wagner, 1994: 315). Wagner argued that the solutions whereby we could transform our maternity structures lay first with women as the principal decision-makers, alongside confident midwives in community-centred maternity and perinatal services where, crucially, the community 'is given the power to monitor and control' those services (1994: 331).

In the intervening two decades we have gained massive understanding in how to achieve Wagner's vision and to dismantle the birth machine. We have also suffered massive setbacks, like the closure of the Albany (Mander and Murphy-Lawless, 2013; Homer *et al.*, 2017). We would argue that these setbacks have stemmed from degraded political and institutional cultures that have run roughshod over commitment, evidence and agency.

The chapters in this section discuss actions which directly challenge seeming powerlessness. These are practical and politically focused undertakings, affirming that women need a secure, caring space to understand themselves as pregnant and new mothers, affirming the pressing need to support midwives and students who long to be there for women but who are currently broken by a broken system. This work has reached deep into communities in multiple ways to raise awareness and to gain concrete change through workshops, theatre, the documentary film, and a country-wide movement for a new law on mandatory inquests.

10

HEALING OURSELVES AS MIDWIVES

Jenny Patterson

The emotional work of midwives

Midwifery is a caring profession. Midwives are passionate and committed individuals who through their working day (and night) strive to provide safe, holistic, nurturing care for women, babies and often their families. The clear majority provide this care within systems beset by significant financial and resource limitations. Midwives are constantly required to balance the external needs and demands of management, regulatory bodies and women, while reconciling within themselves their personal needs, desires, values and drive to fulfil their role in a way which they are satisfied with. Furthermore, midwifery culture is often less than supportive and riddled with bullying (Kirkham, 2007; Gillen *et al.*, 2008, Ellie 2015). External pressures, culture, and personal vision are very often incompatible. This is reflected by the Birth Project Group survey showing the suboptimal lived experience of midwives in fulfilling their role (see Chapters 2 and 4). Much has been written and researched about the 'emotional work' which midwives carry as part of their work (Hunter, 2004), and the negative impact this has on them (Pezaro, 2016).

At this point I would like to consider the following scenario. Imagine there is a large boulder in the middle of the road, just around a corner. The road is not closed as it is passable with care and is an essential connection route. However, many people driving around the corner, do not manage to avoid the boulder (even with a warning), and instead they crash and need treatment. Local budgets do not stretch to removing the boulder, but accidents are happening so often that something needs to be done and there is enough finance to open a small clinic at the side of the road to treat injured people. So, while removing the boulder would stop these accidents, reducing both human and clinic costs, the short-term budget does not allow for this.

This analogy is not perfect, but perhaps it helps to understand that increasing resources and staffing across maternity services alongside measures to develop a holistic, supportive culture in midwifery, would go a long way to improve midwives' experience and health, but this is not yet the reality. On a positive note here, some international nursing models are proving by example that these conditions and constraints can be overcome (Buurtzorg, 2016) and these models are currently being explored within the NHS (RCN, 2016). While speaking out and demanding sustainable improvement in the healthcare system must continue (or campaigning to remove the boulder), in the meantime, many midwives are suffering trauma (Pezaro 2016) and being driven to leave their profession (Campbell, 2016; RCM, 2016b). Walking away, changing jobs, if possible, may be the best and right option for some midwives. But for many it is not a realistic option either financially or in terms of their desire to work with women and to follow a deep calling and identity. In keeping with the above analogy, it is becoming necessary to 'set up the clinic', or in other words enable midwives to find ways to maintain their physical and mental well-being in the healthcare climate.

Resilience within midwifery

This leads to consideration of the term 'resilience'. Resilience can be considered as the ability to withstand or recover quickly from difficult situations: for midwives to continue to practise in the face of the difficulties and adversities they encounter (Crowther *et al.*, 2016). Much has been written about resilience in midwifery (Hunter and Warren, 2013, 2014) and it is argued that midwives should not be required to develop resilience to withstand a damaging and unreasonably pressured working environment (Hunter, 2014; Crowther *et al.*, 2016). Nevertheless, midwives do exist within this environment at present and deserve to be cared for as much as the women they serve. Furthermore, enabling midwives to become well, strong, and resilient, may provide them with the inner resources to experience deep satisfaction with their work, and potentially gain strength, courage, and clarity of vision to call for and drive forward improvements for the benefit of all. So, while we must remain undaunted in our attempts to improve the working environment, it is imperative that midwives are supported in finding realistic, accessible, and effective ways to care for themselves.

What do midwives already do or have access to?

In considering this it must be noted that midwives are already strong and resourceful and many have identified ways of keeping themselves well within the pressures under which they work. There exist suggestions for self-care for midwives (Jackson *et al.*, 2007; Wickham, 2014) as well as resources such as the online module available from *The Practising Midwife* (TPM, 2016). Furthermore, the Royal College of Midwives (RCM) recently launched its 'Caring for You Campaign' (RCM, 2016c).

Introducing another option

In keeping with the role of midwives to provide information based on up-to-date evidence, this chapter now presents a range of self-care practices, rooted in long-standing healing traditions and for which there is a growing body of evidence of their effectiveness. Many of you will have heard of Tai Chi, mindfulness, and acupressure, which are now mainstream terms even if you have never tried them or know much about them. But you have perhaps not heard of 'Capacitar'. Before I tell you more, I feel it would be helpful to tell you a little about my experience as a midwife and why I chose to discover more about Capacitar.

A step back to my journey and experience in midwifery

My journey into midwifery began in 1997, a few weeks after the home birth of my fourth and youngest son. During a conversation with a friend, I experienced an epiphany and knew with almost gut-wrenching certainty that I needed to become a midwife. I spent seven years, while my boys grew, immersed in birth literature and discussions, as well as training via the Scottish Birth Teachers Association (SBTA), now the Birth Educators Course run through the Pregnancy and Parents Centre, Edinburgh, and Doula UK. I was steeped in the social model of midwifery and not only the normality of childbirth, but the incredible power, wonder, and awe of the beautiful, often challenging, and occasionally dangerous process of birth. In 2004, with my boys settled in school and with great family support, I began training as a midwife. From 2007, I developed my working life as a midwife, primarily in independent practice, but also as an NHS bank midwife within both consultant unit and community settings.

The experience was so much more challenging than I had anticipated; not the being with women - but the accommodation of the 'fear', 'guidelines', 'pressures', 'expectations', 'lack of fundamental support', 'bullying', and general lack of being 'looked out for', more being 'gunned for', while trying to offer women holistic, evidence-based, individualised care. This was one thing to experience as a midwife, but to see it meted out to women who did not conform was harrowing. Treading a safe and positive path through this, was, for me, emotionally draining. However, I persisted, even to becoming a Supervisor of Midwives (SoM). Over a period of 15 years I had experienced being in many camps: 'doula', 'hospital midwife', 'community midwife', 'independent midwife', and SoM.

What stood out most, on reflection, was the incredible pressure and fear from within each camp being projected onto those in the other camps. Mistrust was rife, undermining, and most often unfounded. Women caught within this fragmented system found their problems compounded by the widespread mistrust and by inconsistent, and at times unsafe, care and communication.

Why is all this important? Why am I telling you this? Because this frequently broken, fearful, and fragmented system weakens and destroys women's and midwives' confidence. It increases fear, with the potential consequence of poorer, often traumatic outcomes.

I repeatedly rose above or quelled my increasing unease and distress, at one time stopping the car on the way home from a shift to weep uncontrollably. While I am individual in my experience, I now know that I am not unique (see Chapters 4 and 8, Pezaro, 2016). Finally, in December 2012, having reached breaking point again, I had a conversation with a friend, like I did in 1997, which led to following a very new path.

Discovering Capacitar

Many midwives complete training in complementary or alternative medicine (CAM) such as hypnotherapy, aromatherapy, homoeopathy, and herbalism, and practices like yoga, mindfulness and shiatsu. However, while aspects of these were of interest to me, and I completed study days in some, I was never drawn to undertake full training in any. When I read the description of the Capacitar training (Capacitar, 2017a), I was intrigued by the range of modalities included. I must admit that my reasons for completing the training were grounded in my own needs at that time, and not from any desire to offer Capacitar to women or colleagues. However, I quickly realised during the training that Capacitar, while not a magic 'solve it all' solution, was a very effective and realistic option for many people and I could see the potential benefit for childbearing women and midwives.

The development of Capacitar International

During the war and violence in Nicaragua in 1988, an art project leader, Pat Cane, practised daily Tai Chi and acupressure for her own self-care. The community invited her to share this so they could heal the stress of everyday life and their positive experiences led them to share the practices more widely in their extended communities, living out the spirit of Capacitar, which is a Spanish word meaning 'to empower, to bring to life' (Capacitar, 2017b). Capacitar subsequently became the name of what is now a large, non-profit, international organisation, working in over 41 countries around the world. Capacitar collaborates with grassroots communities affected by poverty, violence, trauma and war, and produces materials and manuals in a wide range of languages for both adults and children (Capacitar, 2017c; Capacitar, 2017d).

What does Capacitar involve?

To understand the underlying principles of Capacitar practices, we could discuss energy, life force, meridians, and chakras; terms which may elicit different responses in us depending on our experience or understanding of them. However, human energy flow has been acknowledged by Eastern medicine practices for thousands of years, and has been only more recently recognised in the West, as a result of growing evidence (Rubik, 2008; Guarneri and King, 2015).

We could further talk about brain function, particularly the primitive ancient brain, the limbic brain, the centre of instinct and feeling, and the more recently evolved neocortex, or thinking brain, familiar to midwives in the context of birth and the hormonal physiology of birth and instinctual birthing (Buckley, 2015).

While energy, brain function, and hormones are all relevant (and you are welcome to follow up the references to deepen your knowledge), it is perhaps more helpful to understand simply that our mind, heart, and physical body are driven to work together to move us towards being well and happy (Condon and Cane, 2011). To put it another way, just as midwives understand that women hold deep, inner, instinctual knowledge about birthing their babies, so too do we each have a deep, inner, instinctual knowledge about healing ourselves and maintaining health. When we cannot or will not follow these drives or instincts within us, we can find ourselves hurting, pressured and/or unhappy.

As many of us know, it is rarely possible to use our 'thinking' brain to make a change in our 'feeling' brain; in other words to 'tell' ourselves to 'feel' differently. However, when we engage our bodies, while reflecting in our thoughts, changes can happen in the way we feel. For example, when we are troubled, going for a walk and thinking things through can make us feel differently. The way we engage our bodies and the related impact on our thoughts and feelings have been beautifully described in Amy Cuddy's presentation in the TED talk series (Cuddy, 2012), based on her collaborative research (Carney *et al.*, 2010; Biello, 2017).

What does Capacitar offer?

The Capacitar practices support and enable optimum energy flow, while also creating a connection between our thinking brain and our feeling brain, and both these benefits can result in the person experiencing healing, both physically and mentally. Capacitar offers a wide range of mind/body practices (Condon and Cane, 2011). Some, as mentioned above, are becoming familiar within our culture, such as Tai Chi, acupressure, relaxation visualisations, and mindfulness, with therapies such as Emotional Freedom Technique (EFT) gaining validity as research evidence confirms their effectiveness (Church, 2013; Boath *et al.*, 2017). Others are perhaps less well known at present, such as polarity work or walking labyrinths, while others may not be considered by some to be 'healing' modalities such as dance or prayer.

Developing well-being sessions based on Capacitar

Capacitar International is a grassroots organisation, which emerged from cultures other than ours in Scotland. The stated aim 'to heal ourselves, others and the world', may not feel comfortable to some of us here in Scotland, feeling somewhat 'new age' or 'utopian'. But if we take a moment to look beneath the surface, we can see that regardless of the words we might choose to describe or define the aims of Capacitar, the fact remains that the underlying ethos is to share knowledge and empower others to find ways to care for themselves and those they connect with in life. Looked at this way it becomes more accessible, and potentially acceptable, within our culture.

Over recent years, Eastern practices such as yoga, mindfulness, and Tai Chi, have gained popularity and are to some extent becoming mainstream. It is not a huge leap therefore, to develop well-being sessions that incorporate a range of these practices. What attracted me to Capacitar was the simplicity and accessibility of the practices, requiring nothing more than a willingness to take part and an openness to learn. The level at which each is offered is easy to learn without intense physical or mental discipline. This was extremely refreshing, as it meant they could be incorporated into busy and pressured lives, without adding another source of stress.

In exploring how I might share this work, I first needed to consider how to present it, so that it felt accessible and welcoming to as many people as possible. Following completion of the year long training, I began offering regular well-being sessions and workshops in Edinburgh, based on the Capacitar practices. Many sessions were open to everyone, while others were specifically offered for pregnant women or new mothers, or directed towards midwives, student midwives, doulas, and others involved in the care of childbearing women. Beyond Edinburgh, further workshops for midwives took place in Dublin; the University of West of Scotland (Ayr and Paisley); Southern General Hospital, Glasgow; Ninewells Hospital, Dundee; and the Ayrshire maternity unit. I have provided breakout workshops at the Queens Nursing Institute of Scotland (QNIS) annual conference 2016, as well as the QNIS training programme in March 2017 and for a Scottish cohort of Parkinson's specialist nurses in 2016.

A typical workshop would contain a mixture of the gentle Korean stretching exercises, known as Pal Dan Gum as well as some gentle Tai Chi. There would be time to sit quietly and focus on the breath, perhaps using different techniques to deepen the breath or maintain awareness and mindfulness. A core practice, from an ancient form of acupressure known as Jin Shin Jyutsu, involves gently but firmly holding our fingers, one at a time. This is an incredibly simple yet effective way to reduce the intensity of strong, possibly overwhelming emotions (Figure 10.1). An introduction to the self-use of EFT is yet another core practice (Capacitar, 2017c). Note that the level at which these would be taught in a session is safe for people of all ages to use. Individuals are always encouraged to listen to their own bodies, especially with any of the movement exercises, and only do what feels comfortable for them.

Evaluation of the sessions

In recognition of the importance, and indeed the NHS requirement, to evaluate and measure outcomes and feedback from sessions, I explored ways to do this. Initially, an evaluation sheet was provided at the end of sessions and workshops,

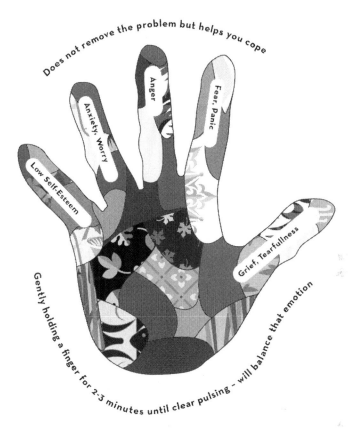

FIGURE 10.1 Postcard given out at wellbeing sessions, showing instructions for the fingerholds

© OnlyConnect Health 2015

enabling feedback on the quality of the sessions in terms of information and length, along with each person's initial response to the techniques presented. However, it could not measure the subsequent impact on the well-being of the person, and so I searched for a way to do this. I was particularly drawn to the Warwick and Edinburgh Mental Wellbeing Scale (WEMWBS) (Warwick Medical School, 2015; Stewart-Brown *et al.*, 2011), which utilises 14 Likert-scale questions, because the 14 questions in the adult scale are positively framed. As required by the designers, Frances Taggart and Sarah Stewart-Brown, I sought and received permission to use this scale within my sessions. However, I realised that for it to be useful, I needed to have a measure on the scale before and after experiencing the sessions and this was not realistic after only one session. Aside from one-off workshops, the main weekly events were drop-in sessions. Some people regularly attended the weekly sessions while others came to a few, often in an ad hoc way depending on other life commitments. Often new folk would drop in for a week or two. Not knowing who would be there from one week to the next made it difficult to collect 'before' and 'after' measures of well-being. Also, because new people would attend, it was often best to keep the sessions focused only on the basic techniques, not progressing unless those present were already familiar with the basics. This was limiting not only in terms of evaluation but in terms of progress for the regular attendees. To address this, I ran a few fixed blocks of four- or six-week sessions. These enabled people to discover the basic techniques, practice these weekly, and experience further advanced techniques. Fifteen people started these sessions and 11 people completed them. While it was not possible to find out why people stopped coming, it must be presumed that the sessions did not feel right for them, although it may have been other life circumstances that intervened. Eleven people consented to completing the WEMWBS prior to the first session and at the end of the final session after either four or six weeks, depending on the group. The WEMWBS from the first session were completed and returned to me at the first session, and so participants did not reread these when they completed the second one at the end of the sessions. The score levels were calculated.

The WEMWBS has 14 questions, all beginning with 'In the last two weeks I have been feeling', followed by a series of descriptors, and for each question there is the option of selecting a level:

1   not at all
2   rarely
3   some of the time
4   often
5   all the time.

Total scores were calculated as recommended by WEMWBS (Putz et al., 2012) and an NHS scoring system (NHS Choices, 2011) was used to categorise the total scores for each participant, at each time point (box 10.1).

Box 10.1 Total score levels

Scoring system	No. at start
0–32 very low well-being scale	0
32–40 below average well-being scale	2 [1 moved to above average (+29), 1 moved to average (+18)]
40–59 average well-being score	9 [9 remained average (2 same score, 7 increased scores)]
59–70 above average well-being score	0

Nine people had an increase in their overall score by an average of 12 points. Two people had the same score. No one had a reduced overall score. For most people, their rating increased in most categories, or at least stayed the same in others. For two people the increase was mostly by two or three levels. Four people rated a drop in only one category out of 14, one person rated a drop in four categories (Table 10.1). There were no drops of more than one level.

While this is a very small sample, it is nonetheless illustrative of the potential benefit of the well-being practices offered by Capacitar.

TABLE 10.1 Changes in scores for each category on WEMWBS following 4–6 sessions

	No. of people whose score was		
Category	Up	Same	Down
I have (been/feeling)			
optimistic about the future	6	5	0
useful	6	5	0
relaxed	6	4	1
interested in others	7	4	0
energy to spare	7	3	1
dealing with problems well	7	4	0
thinking clearly	5	5	1
good about myself	9	2	0
close to others	5	5	1
confident	7	4	0
make up my own mind	4	5	2
loved	4	6	1
interested in new things	4	7	0
cheerful	7	3	1

From the assessment sheets, there is qualitative data about individual experiences, the clear majority of which were positive. A few were more constructive than positive, but none were negative (Table 10.2).

Summary of findings

The WEMWBS scores and evaluation feedback showed that the Capacitar practices were not only well received and enjoyed, but had a positive impact on the emotional well-being of those who took part. Reflecting on this, along with the 41 years of positive experience and assessment within Capacitar International, it appears that these practices may be realistic and viable self-care options for midwives.

Conclusion

Midwives are passionate about and committed to providing optimum care for women and babies, but the context and environment in which they provide this

TABLE 10.2 Feedback received from sessions and workshops

Below is a selection of the positive feedback

'I have used some of the techniques taught and already feel better'

'I intend to do it regularly have really enjoyed the sessions'

'Teaching very good, well communicated'

'Has been very helpful, beyond the techniques, understanding the importance of setting aside 5 or 10 minutes each day to relax and clear'

'When I use stuff from Capacitar it is always beneficial'

'I didn't know what to expect, but now I know I really liked it and will use it'

'Vocabulary and instructions were great really simple'

'Nice to have some alternative healing methods'

'Really enjoyed this session and will recommend to others'

'Really simple techniques not too complex at all'

'Very useful, felt very relaxed after the workshop'

'Not sure of what to expect, at the conclusion I felt this was a rewarding experience'

'A really useful, gentle and enjoyable workshop'

'Really interesting opened my eyes to new ideas'

'Wonderful! Unknown territory before the session'

'I've enjoyed it very much; have gained so much, feeling empowered and ready to conquer the stuff I needed to. Feeling much calmer and relaxed'

'Extremely beneficial'

'It was just right – you're great at explaining things'

'It has really helped me overcome some major hurdles and I have been recommending to others'

Constructive feedback

'I would like to have a small handout so I can retrieve the techniques at home'★

'I have arthritis and found some of the exercises difficult'

'One or two more sessions would be good'

'Capacitar is not a name known so may be a marketing challenge'

★ Handouts now exist as well as a short DVD of the exercises

care is beset with many pressures and limitations. Great demands are placed on midwives and result in many midwives experiencing stress and/or trauma and a growing number choose to leave the profession. These systemic problems may remain unresolved for some time, yet there is an urgent need to enable midwives to care for themselves and retain their strength, vision and passion for caring for women, which in turn may enable them to further the drive towards systemic improvements in maternity services. Capacitar International offers a range of practical self-care practices, which are effective and safe as well as easy to learn, use and pass on to others. For those who feel drawn to any, or indeed many, of these practices I would urge you to consider undertaking the Capacitar training, which is very manageable, even around full-time work.

11

CREATING A COMMUNITY OF SUPPORT FOR PREGNANT WOMEN AND NEW MOTHERS

Nadine Edwards and Bridget Sheeran

What support do pregnant women and new mothers need?

This chapter considers how two unique grassroots projects grew out of women's own experiences of being unable to gain vital information and support which they needed from the maternity services in Scotland and Ireland during their pregnancies and after birth. It shows how women learned from each other, developed greater knowledge about the context of birth, increased trust in their own bodies, gained confidence in their abilities to be capable mothers and developed a strong, supportive and lasting network during the early years of parenting.

The context

The most recent maternity policy review in Scotland (Scottish Government, 2017) recommends building maternity care upon relationships between women and midwives by providing continuity of carer throughout the childbearing journey. This has been shown to provide the safest care (Sandall, Coxon *et al.*, 2016) and to work for women and midwives (Homer *et al.*, 2017). It has the potential to increase women's confidence as pregnant women and new mothers and to build on and strengthen community networks (Leap, 2010). This is exactly the organisation of care needed for women and midwives to maintain genuine agency and build on their knowledge and skills together. But there remains an enormous gulf between current maternity provision and the transformational possibilities of this aspirational policy. In Ireland, the maternity strategy (Ireland Department of Health and Children, 2016) aims to place women at the centre of the service and to provide continuity of care. The strategy is the first of its kind and has taken 70 years to bring about, yet it fails to properly address the support and relationships needed within midwifery, and the quality community-based services that would support women's greater agency (Wood, 2017). Formidable challenges lie ahead for both countries.

With exemplary exceptions, most women report that midwives are trying to do their very best but are too busy to do much more than provide routine care during pregnancy. Antenatal appointments tend to follow a set content, depending on the number of weeks pregnant the woman is, with little room for deviation. Some women report being unable to get the emotional reassurance they need, or to have detailed discussions about their specific circumstances. After birth, especially if they have had obstetric interventions, some women struggle to recover physically and emotionally; they struggle with breastfeeding and suffer from postnatal depression, exhaustion and isolation. Under the current regime, midwives are less and less able to provide anything more than limited postnatal visits in the UK while in Ireland some units provide no postnatal visits. Local services which do provide home visits limit these to three or four. Again with notable exceptions, concrete support through the statutory systems currently in place is too often prescriptive or haphazard.

The broader policies and practices over the last decades that have tried to improve support for families and reduce the impact of growing inequalities have all too often been seen as tools of surveillance and monitoring rather than as being supportive, and have embedded the notion of the professional as expert rather than building on the strengths of families and communities (Murphy Lawless *et al.*, unpublished, Ormston *et al.*, 2014, www.scotland.gov.uk/Resource/0044/00444851.pdf).

However, where initiatives have been developed by women, or by women and midwives working together to support women's stated needs, they have attracted positive feedback and have provided a range of benefits (Armstrong *et al.*, 2006; Garlick, 2016; Nicoll *et al.*, 2005; Reed, 2016).

The initiatives described below draw on similar approaches. They are local attempts to care for pregnant women, new mothers and their families, and to develop strong networks that support families well beyond the initiatives themselves. They also attempt to provide information and support for women to feel more confident, exert greater agency, and make decisions about their own bodies and babies.

The Pregnancy and Parents Centre, Edinburgh

In the 1970s, I (Nadine) encountered a lack of information and support within maternity services for my decisions about how and where to have my babies, and an outdated, prescriptive approach to caring for a new baby. With this in mind, I started a small informal group for pregnant women in their homes (or mine) in 1985. It met once a week to do some 'relaxation', 'breathing' and 'body work' and to talk. Setting up these groups was an attempt to provide a safe space for pregnant women to come together to share their aspirations, knowledge and experiences and develop the confidence to be able to question some of the then (entirely unresearched and potentially damaging) routine practices of the 1980s: continuous electronic fetal monitoring, lying down during labour and birth, episiotomies, and syntometrine for the delivery of the placenta. These are all practices which women increasingly questioned and resisted. Over time, research supported our concerns about the damaging consequences of these practices when used routinely. What was clear from these first informal groups was that, whatever their individual views, women wanted to be involved in decisions about their labours and births. Having created this space, we read the research and I started a library of reliable books about pregnancy and birth based on good research. We learned from and supported each other to negotiate the increasingly fragmented, medicalised and centralised maternity care system.

Through the open discussions with tea and cake at the end of the 'body work', women often found that they had views and experiences in common. An informal, supportive network began to develop. Women wanted to come back to meet after their babies were born, and so the weekly postnatal groups started. Then there came baby music, baby massage and postnatal yoga. A local AIMS (Association for Improvements in the Maternity Services) group flowed from this, as did a home-birth support group. Alliances were formed with midwives from the Association of Radical Midwives. A birth educators training course materialised in the early 1990s. A charity was formed (initially the Birth Resource Centre and now the Pregnancy and Parents Centre) and the groups moved from my home to a community centre before receiving funding from a small local trust so that it could rent its own premises. Influencing maternity services is challenging, but over the years the Centre has raised awareness about pregnancy, birth and parenting within its community; maintained a presence on the local Maternity Services Liaison Committee; submitted papers to local Health Boards and the Scottish Office; contributed to national policy groups and consultations; and posted research findings on its website and Facebook page.

Since its modest beginnings in 1985, the Centre has grown far more than expected. It is now located in a two-storey building in central Edinburgh surrounded by garages and warehouses. It provides groups, workshops, one-to-one and drop-in sessions, often seven days and many evenings per week. There is yoga for pregnancy; birth preparation for women and partners; and dads to be; birth choices; new arrivals for those new to Edinburgh without family or friends; support for mothers with very young babies; yoga for parents and babies; baby massage; music for parents with babies, toddlers and pre-school children; breast-feeding support; counselling; homeopathy; craniosacral therapy; birth educators training courses; evening talks, conferences and more. It has a multinational research group, a website and a Facebook page, a well-stocked library, and a permanent display of donated maternity wear, baby clothes and cloth nappies. The Centre is managed by a group of voluntary trustees, most of whom have used the Centre in the past, supported by three members of staff, as well as facilitators, practitioners and volunteers. All in all, over 500 people who form a community around the Centre come through the doors each week, and parents who came to the groups as long ago as 25–30 years still meet.

The Centre receives a small amount of funding for some of its drop-in groups but mainly supports itself through a flexible payment or donation system, fundraising events (nearly new sales, evening talks), donations and hiring out rooms, birth pools and TENS (transcutaneous electrical nerve stimulation) machines. It endeavours to welcome all, irrespective of their economic circumstances. It focuses on building self-esteem, inspiring confidence and encouraging friendships. Our belief is that straightforward birth followed by breastfeeding usually provides the best start for parents and babies, but there is no dogma. Women are welcomed back with their babies to tell us their stories whatever their decisions and however their births have unfolded.

Over the years, women have told us that they feel safe at the Centre, even when they feel vulnerable. They value sharing their experiences, learning from each other, feeling respected, being part of a supportive network, held, and encouraged through pregnancy and new motherhood (Armstrong *et al.*, 2006; Edwards, 2014). As one pregnant woman who is a lone parent recently said:

> *This is such an **amazing** resource. I always feel so much better after I've been here and there'll be the Monday* [drop-in group for new mothers] *... It makes me think – 'I can do this, it's going to be alright'.*

After having her baby, this woman sent the following:

> *It was an amazingly supportive environment. I cannot tell you how valuable those classes were for me. They were magically relaxing but also an absolute pleasure, which I looked forward to every week. It's very hard to express just how much those classes and the PPC have meant to me – but I'm so grateful, plan to remain an avid PPC'er and to hopefully contribute in lots of ways over the coming years.*

Many women tell us that they feel more confident as their pregnancies progress – more confident in their bodies and their abilities to birth their babies, more confident that they have the information they need, and more confident that they will be able to mother their babies in their own ways. In other words they develop greater trust in themselves and their decisions. The prenatal sessions have been described as 'life changing' and the postnatal groups have been described as a 'lifeline'. One mother of three said that she had tried many different groups and places, and the moment she set foot in the Centre she felt at home. Often it is described as a 'haven', especially by student midwives and midwives who visit the Centre or who work, volunteer, or complete a placement with us.

BabyTalk, Skibbereen, West Cork, Ireland

In 1999, I (Bridget) took time off from my independent midwifery practice where I offered complete care to rural women and their babies from early pregnancy until six weeks postnatally; this was my response to the realities of women living in a rural area over 80 kilometres of pot-holed winding roads from the nearest hospital maternity services. I was having my fourth baby and my third home birth in this rural area.

At the time, outside of my own practice and the practices of a handful of other home-birth midwives, there was virtually no preparation for birth, no information about recovery after birth or the new-born period and no access to midwives from the hospital for the mothers in West Cork planning hospital births. Women primarily relied on sometimes questionable information from family or their GP. This remains the current situation if they do not opt for a self-employed community midwife who can give continuity of care and support throughout pregnancy, birth and the postnatal period.

Women are told to consult professionals and not to ask their mothers for advice. At the same time, the so-called prescriptive version of 'normality', promoted to women by professionals then and now, leaves so much to chance and reflects a disturbing lack of relevant knowledge and information. Mothers get the impression that they need to become a 'professional mother' to get it right, endlessly reading articles and popular books, yet the health professional may be advising approaches which are not necessarily based on evidence (such as giving antibiotics for mastitis, when 80 per cent of mastitis is non-infective – this still happens in Skibbereen). Local GPs and hospital midwives are not readily available for most queries and much time is used by women to get reassurance about often media-generated fears of dangerous and improbable diseases, or of doing something drastically wrong. This fear-mongering is part of the expanding sense that pregnancy is only healthy and normal in retrospect and that by virtue of becoming pregnant a woman now faces a wide range of innumerable 'risks' for which ongoing measuring and testing in pregnancy becomes routine, with no preparation or discussion about what to expect or why a woman is being tested. This approach severely undermines women, who are left with uncertainty and doubt, very little agency (to refuse testing of any sort is to be viewed as an 'irresponsible mother'), but who carry full responsibility for all outcomes.

I decided to see how I could meet women with their babies. I knew it was difficult, and it was only because I was a midwife that I had an inkling of who was having a baby in my community. As I also knew, women in Ireland who plan hospital births have no access to self-employed community midwives like myself and no easy access to other local women for support in pregnancy, or postnatally, compared to women who plan a home birth with a self-employed community midwife. I wanted to reach these women and offer a place for them to find up-to-date, reliable information about birthing, feeding a baby and recovering from birth. With no opportunity to learn comprehensively about birth and mothering during their pregnancies from the hospital services, women often relied on outmoded views about birth and babies, supplemented by the latest alarming stories reported in the media.

I started BabyTalk in my own home, with my new baby, and brought local guests in to teach baby massage, yoga postures and relaxation methods such as ginger compresses (the best-kept secret!). My need to reach more women outside of the home-birth circle led me into Skibbereen town to facilitate BabyTalk. It needed to be free for women. This was achieved initially through the local Bantry Integrated Development Group in order to keep BabyTalk independent. Subsequently it was funded by the national Department of Social, Community and Family Affairs which led (unexpectedly for me) to the Health Board funding the 'project', bringing BabyTalk very much into the realm of public health. I was told that funds were diverted from family planning and later Mother and Toddler Group-funding to support the very low costs of BabyTalk which, if true, raised questions about exactly how much women's needs as mothers were valued in West Cork, if a mothering support group was traded off against other crucial needs of mothers of young children.

The venues changed unexpectedly from time to time but all were selected on the basis of being accessible for those walking or driving and having no stairs, so that buggies could be wheeled in. There were difficulties with inappropriate settings, such as one in a clinical 'health' environment with a very noisy vending machine full of sugary drinks, cheap sweets and chocolate bars. The current venue is the Family Resource Centre, Skibbereen.

Each BabyTalk session was two hours in length, with a series of eight weekly sessions for any one group. Drawing on my experience as a community midwife, I welcomed each woman and her baby into the group, fostering a non-judgemental atmosphere, enabling everyone to meet each other, and inviting everyone to share their names (ensuring that there was no expectation to remember these) and where they lived. This made it possible to find new neighbours and to open up car sharing for transport - an important element in a rural area with no regular public transport. I would open the session with the question: 'Would anyone like to share their fondest memory of the birth – it can be the first few moments, or up to six weeks later – whatever brings a positive memory?'

In the first group I ran, although women in Skibbereen rarely complained openly about their births, invariably there was a negative feel to their exchanges about their births; or they said nothing until a woman mentioned some specific detail of the birth, like seeing the shock of her baby's hair (usually a home-birth woman). I eventually found out that this was because the majority of women in the group had had either a surgical birth or an induction, forceps or ventouse birth. I was deeply disturbed by this and shocked that women assumed that these interventions were normal, that caesarean birth was 'abnormal' and that home birth was illegal.

From that moment on I set about facilitating BabyTalk to help women to talk about birth with each other, to acknowledge the best intentions of midwives working in the maternity services, while at the same time being able to question why the services were so poor in supporting normal healthy labours and birthing. Some women realised by talking to other women that they had been coerced into interventions and were able to consider how to do things differently next time. This maintained their self-esteem while encouraging exploration and questions that I could then answer if asked.

The lack of birth preparation was painful to witness. Women were unable to use their bodies, minds or voices to their advantage because birth was not talked about and it was assumed that doctors knew best. This also applied to breastfeeding. There was little understanding about new-born needs or breastfeeding initiation and bottle feeding was totally accepted in the community. This created a barrier to breastfeeding for more than a few weeks (even though the first La Leche League group in the south of Ireland started in Skibbereen).

I knew that women needed to hear about breastfeeding and to see other women breastfeeding, so that new ideas about feeding could be shared. Some women chose to breastfeed their next baby because they saw how convenient it was and found bottle feeding was not what they had expected, with an unsettled and crying baby and the extra work of sterilising.

The deeper support within the group developed quickly, and over the years attitudes changed as most women knew someone who had told them 'not to miss BabyTalk'. The group became sought after and far more open to more intimate discussions. Women who might not normally have socialised together became friends and were so interested in other mothers' opinions about soothers, nappies, rashes, baby nails, cradle cap, green stools, dealing with well-meaning but unwanted advice, sunscreens, going back to work, expressing milk, the importance of attachment, slings, stress-management of christenings or naming ceremonies, weaning foods, crying babies, sibling jealousy, and sleep patterns. Women felt safe and had a sense of contributing to something positive, something that worked. This matters at very profound levels in reducing isolation and creating new spaces for mothers in the wider community.

From time to time over the years fathers came to the group. This proved to be challenging as, although they were always welcomed, the women shared that their presence inhibited what they might talk about – for instance, the first period after birth, contraception, the first lovemaking, the need for sleep, and even the need not to be touched at times. One dad was the local postman who delivered post to the venue so he used to pop his head in to say 'Hello!'

Being in a rural setting, husbands and partners travel huge distances for work, so days are very long for new mothers with families far away. Women have felt very isolated, even with a car, so BabyTalk was invaluable. The sessions have received consistently positive feedback:

> So great to actually get out of the house and meet other mums.
>
> Lovely to hear what other mums are doing.
>
> Great to meet other mothers, and realise that you are not going crazy.
>
> I was feeling isolated and like I was re-inventing the wheel, before BabyTalk.
>
> Thank you for the wealth of information, for giving advice, support and ideas without making me feel inadequate as a mother (as unwelcome advice can do).

I feel confident and self-assured now in my new job and am loving it [being a mother].

Just helpful hints and the way we were helped with our confidence, facilitator Bridget was brill.

Since 1999, BabyTalk has reached about 500 families in the local area. It is unique, free to women, and supported by Public Health Nurses who contribute sessions on hazards in the home, choking, and postnatal exercises. Access to midwifery experience and advice is not the rule in the maternity services and postnatal care is, as we have already stated above, almost non-existent. The essence of BabyTalk lies in women learning from women. Making life-long friends (some groups are still meeting regularly themselves ten years or more later) is a strong dimension of this. BabyTalk is not a class or a therapy but the outcome is women learning to make their own decisions, learning that it is safe to connect outside of their usual worlds, learning how to find the positive, building and bonding with their community in a non-judgemental manner, and setting up useful local services for their communities through the networks they build up. Since BabyTalk's inception, Skibbereen has increased its activities about town for women and babies. Baby yoga, sling share and rent schemes, breastfeeding support, and information sharing are just some of the women's groups that have formed.

The supportive, open and non-judgemental approach fostered in BabyTalk was particularly evident when teenage and single mothers were honoured, because the other women realised how hard it must be for them, and recognised how well they were coping with challenging and often stressful living circumstances.

BabyTalk celebrates women and shows them (without telling them) different ways that they might interact with their babies (hence the name I gave it, BabyTalk) through demonstrations and of course discussion to help women to learn skills for raising a healthy family. The population in and around Skibbereen is about 2,000 and BabyTalk has impacted on most families in the area over the course of its eighteen successful years. The smallness of Skibbereen has enabled its success alongside a sense that it can do its work below the official radar, not least because so little is otherwise available from statutory services. So BabyTalk is an 'Irish solution to an Irish problem', as we might say.

Maintaining and developing community projects around pregnancy and new motherhood

These groups and community-building around new motherhood is very context-dependent. Expanding and integrating these sorts of community initiatives while maintaining women's agency and voices so that they can determine what their needs are can be challenging. For example, the Pregnancy and Parents Centre has limitations because of a lack of statutory funding, recognition and support, and thus it can reach only so far. Over the years, local midwives, health visitors and GPs have recognised the benefits of its work and recommend the Centre to women, but we need small community hubs of this kind in many localities. We need ways to support initiatives like BabyTalk in Skibereen in many other localities in Ireland. Many women using the Pregnancy and Parents Centre remark on how lucky they are as there is no other Centre like it in Scotland. To develop such community hubs in partnership with the Scottish NHS and other services would need a concerted effort by health practitioners and statutory services to engage with the community and trust the community to determine what it needs. While there are leaders in this respect (Macintosh, 2011), there remains a reticence to engage: we are rarely consulted about antenatal education when changes are planned; we were not asked to make a submission to the group conducting the most recent Scottish Maternity Review, and it was impossible to gain NHS engagement for a research project planned to support young, pregnant women.

BabyTalk has faced similar challenges, especially keeping hold of a suitable venue. Further afield in County Cork in Bantry and Dunmanway, local community family resource centres have hosted BabyTalk sessions. However, these sessions have not been led by community self-employed midwives but by Public Health Nurses with a remit much more in line with the policies of the Health Service Executive which runs the Irish health services nationally. This has created a different dynamic where the woman-to-woman learning is diluted. While the information imparted by the Public Health Nurses may have some value, it is almost as if well-meaning professionals find the set policies irresistible and take up a didactic rather than a reflexive teaching position, making it the opposite of a partnership. This approach is less likely to recognise the value of woman-to-woman learning. It undermines the very process that enables new mothers to grow in confidence and strength, so that they try out different solutions and find the solution that fits best within their family, as was the hallmark of the original BabyTalk sessions.

These two initiatives, the Pregnancy and Parents Centre in Edinburgh and BabyTalk in Skibbereen, point to the crucial importance of communities themselves taking on the task of creating and sustaining spaces at the local level for pregnant and new mothers, which women can define and develop in line with their needs and where their evolving understanding and knowledge have transformative potential.

12

PERFORMING THE REVOLUTION, CREATING A COUNTER-NARRATIVE ON BIRTH IN IRELAND

Kate Harris

Daughters of the Revolution is a theatre performance drawn from the lived experiences of women and midwifery students within the Irish maternity services. It was created both as a response to those experiences and as an invitation to health care practitioners and the public to start a conversation to find ways the maternity services could work better for everyone.

The play was developed in the context of Irish maternity services, where outcomes for women and their babies are average at best and where a climate of powerlessness acutely affects women and midwives alike. It is a system where medical authority is foremost and where women are constrained to respond from a position of vulnerability, where their embodied knowledge and the knowledge of their midwife advocates is not acknowledged or valued (Morgan, 1998: 92). As a theatre maker using the Theatre of the Oppressed to make theatre for social change, I was uniquely placed to respond to my own experience of birth within the hospital system.

Theatre of the Oppressed was developed by the Brazilian theatre practitioner Augusto Boal. Theatre of the Oppressed has been used in working with communities throughout the world over the last 40 years. It creates a platform for marginalised people in society to voice their experiences and to rehearse ways to make lasting social change. Theatre of the Oppressed techniques have been utilised in schools, prisons, hospitals, in conflict situations, and with marginalised rural and urban communities (Boal, 1992: 241).

Theatre of the Oppressed is concerned with disrupting the dominant narrative. Dominant narratives within a society are created through the 'interacting social, economic, political, and symbolic structures' (Morgan, 1998: 86). The dominant narrative on birth in Ireland is one of medical authority, where scientific knowledge is privileged over the embodied knowledge of women and the embodied practice of midwives. When confronted with a dominant narrative of medical authority that devalued and dismissed me, I did not want to make a complaint; I wanted to make a play.

Daughters of the Revolution was developed over a period of four years, using Theatre of the Oppressed methodologies in drama workshops to research the experiences of women using the maternity services and midwifery students training in the services. In these workshops, participants articulated the contested and hierarchical nature of knowledge in relation to pregnancy and birth, and the conflict between embodied and empirical ways of knowing. Based on research from the drama workshops, and informed by many conversations with professionals working in the field of maternity policy, *Daughters of the Revolution* uses theatre to deconstruct the dominant narrative of medical authority through reconstructing the experience of hospital-based maternity in an explicitly theatrical context.

In March 2016, this work led to a revolutionary performance in Dublin.

On three nights, over 120 people, including hospital obstetricians, midwives, academics, midwifery students, birth-choice activists, and members of the public came together, in one room, to see *Daughters of the Revolution*, a play about women's experience of maternity in Ireland.

Daughters of the Revolution is a theatrical provocation, here defined as a challenge to the dominant narrative of medical authority. Drawing on the lived experiences of women within the Irish maternity services and student midwives, the play links the personal to the political. It affirms women's experiences and explores the power dynamic underlying the maternity services.

The intention of the performance was firstly to bring women's stories about birth – stories which often remain hidden – and place these stories centre-stage. These stories created a counter-narrative to the dominant discourse by directly embodying the experiences of women and midwives. Secondly, the public performance of the play sought to start a wider conversation on maternity in Ireland, through dialogue with health care professionals. The post-show discussion between the audience and a panel of experts represented a range of perspectives on maternity in Ireland, including obstetric consultants, midwives, doulas, academics, and maternity-service users. Finally, *Daughters of the Revolution* was created in hope that, by bringing people together to share their different stories, perspectives, and experiences, a new approach to improve the maternity services might emerge.

Daughters of the Revolution performances created a context for the different players to come together, face-to-face, in a shared theatre experience. The uncathected nature of theatre provided a neutral space for individuals to witness the collective experience of women in the maternity services. It levelled resistant professional hierarches so that when audiences came to the post-show discussion there was an equality of voice to start speaking about what could change to improve birth for women and health care professionals. This performance successfully challenged the dominant discourse of medical authority, and with the different perspectives on maternity brought together in one room, it modelled a process of dialogue where women, their partners and families, doulas, academics, midwives, and consultants could speak with equality of voice – and be heard.

The personal is political: Deconstructing the dominant narrative of medical authority through performance

As feminists, we know that political action requires building groups and group knowledge. We must first be able to see ourselves, to tell our stories and connect them to the larger struggle. 'Theatre is the art of looking at ourselves', of making the invisible visible (Boal, 1992: xxx); theatre performance can embody and transmit our stories in ways that ignite the imagination of our communities.

It began with one story, my story, about a woman isolated and enraged with a maternity hospital that refused to listen. When I began to tell my story, I found I was far from alone. Through my telling, I tapped into an underground river of women's stories. Stories that are shared in the private spaces where new mothers gather, at the kitchen table, in playgroups, in waiting rooms. Stories of a lack, an absence: of choice, of respect, of listening, of care.

The gathering of stories was deeply political. These hidden narratives revealed the lines of power and showed that many women struggle to be at the centre of our experience in maternity and birth. These stories needed a form that would acknowledge women's experiences and create a space for women to have an equal voice on how maternity services serve women. These stories needed a platform where they could reach the wider community and inspire change. This was the work I knew how to do.

Between 2013 and 2015 I worked with women who had experienced the maternity services in Ireland and with midwifery students from Trinity College Dublin. I led a series of drama workshops, using Theatre of the Oppressed techniques to create a theatrical language to embody our shared experiences of birth within the hospital setting. By gathering and affirming women's and midwives' stories, we re-contextualised the experience of birth into a theatre performance, creating a counter-narrative, one that was shaped outside the dominant discourse and yet maintained a dialogue with it. In the workshops with women who had used the maternity services, we looked for common threads of experience that would form the basis of our theatrical language. Using still images, tableau, sound, and movement we developed a lexicon to convey the essential lived experiences of women.

One of the most powerful images from the workshop showed a woman physically separated from her birth experience, a voiceless observer at the edge of the scene, while monitors and charts claimed the attention of the medical team. When the creator of the tableau was asked to show the opposite of that experience, she slowly took the other two women by the hand so that one supported her from behind, and the other faced her holding one hand, while the other rested on the woman's stomach and met her gaze.

Theatre allows people to draw on the deepest level of emotional experience, and creates the critical distance to recognise the framework we are all embedded in (Salverson, 1994: 158). Women saw themselves in each other's stories and, importantly, saw themselves with a degree of emotional distance that enabled them to look more critically at the environment that the story took place in. The use of drama gave us tools to step outside our usual roles in the maternity service and examine our own experiences from the perspective of other women, rather than through the lens of medical authority.

Medical authority is reinforced at every level of society: through television and newspaper representations of birth; exerted informally by well-meaning friends and family; and through individual interactions with medical practitioners (Morgan, 1998: 95). As women, we internalise this notion of the dominance of medical authority. Women become alienated from their bodies at an early point in the maternity process, taking on the medical perspective that we are unreliable witnesses when it comes to our own bodies.

Through the act of performing our experiences, we clearly articulated the nature of the roles women must perform to satisfy society's requirements for 'responsible pregnancy' (Morgan, 1998: 95). We confronted the false binary opposition between a woman's experience and medically defined safety. In the workshops, women showed how failures of care were seen as the price paid to be safe, and that there were frightening potential consequences to the resistance of medical authority. Refusal to consent to procedures was quickly labelled as 'lack of compliance' (Morgan, 1998: 92). By recognising the performative role constructed for women by the dominant narrative, we deconstructed the narrative of authoritative empirical knowledge and reasserted our authority over our embodied knowledge by authoring our own lived reality.

During the workshop process, we were joined by student midwives and a researcher in the sociology of maternity. Their experiences furthered our understanding of the power dynamics within maternity hospitals. I remember two momentous pieces, devised by the women and the students to show the lines of power in the hospital. The first showed a consultant whose every small movement was amplified by the midwife and transmitted to the woman, resulting in any movement by the consultant sending the woman careering around the room. The second was a piece that showed caesarean deliveries as an assembly line, performed with shouts of 'NEXT!' every few seconds, whereby everyone would change places and start again. These images were shocking and yet they were a performance of our collective lived experience. Through the abstract representation of the maternity hospital, we immediately recognised the emotional reality of our experiences and found elements of our theatrical language that could speak to a wider audience.

In 2014 and 2015, I had the opportunity to work again with midwifery students through drama workshops. I had found their perspective and understandings of the maternity services an essential part of the story thus far. With the midwifery students, I had a group that were not the object of medical scrutiny but uniquely placed to observe it.

In 2014, having been focused on the narrative from women's perspective as care receivers, I was unprepared for the grim struggle the students faced in the hospitals. In a series of physical representations and short scenes, the students showed their struggle to support women in conditions of unstable levels of care. They showed their experiences of being expected to make up for understaffing or to take the blame. The students represented in role-plays the toxic hierarchical system they experienced on placement, where each sub-section within the hospital protected their area of influence and enforced the pecking order through systematic bullying. It was a bleak picture. These students were trained to support women, and understood the value of women's embodied knowledge, but found themselves utterly unsupported in offering the level of care they had been trained to deliver.

The drama workshops with the midwifery students in 2015 showed the same chaotic environment within the hospitals. The students recreated scenes where chronic understaffing left them alone, and without support, to face care situations with which they were not qualified to deal. The students explored how they negotiated the competing knowledges of midwives and doctors and the different understandings of how care should be delivered. Through these scenes we worked to deconstruct the hospital environment and found ways to represent the students from a position of strength. The students showed different ways they could step out of the dominant narrative to support women, without taking on all the freight of an overstrained hospital system. We created a theatrical language of still strength, of holding one's ground in contested territory, of being anchored through being fully present in care for women.

The narrative around the process of birth is contested territory. Hospitals construct one version, women in care another:

> our experiences are constructed by obstetrics and both their theories and practices ... The weight of our disturbing and uncomfortable personal experiences within this dominant male institution pulls at us to challenge that appearance of normality but we are very often left without effective tools to do so.
>
> (Murphy-Lawless, 1998: 32)

Women and midwives feel the pull to challenge socially constructed roles based on accepted authorities. This is the dominant narrative. By constructing a different narrative through the theatrical performance of embodied knowledge, we gain the tools to create a framework to question the nature of those constructed roles and authority. We moved from a place where we were acted upon, to one where we acted and reasserted our power and authority over our experiences.

The process of weaving together the threads of theatrical language discovered in the workshop space with stories from the wider community created the fabric of the play script. The material for the performance was explicitly grounded in the lived experience of women and midwifery students acting within the maternity services. This counter-narrative sought to directly challenge and interrogate the dominant narrative of empirical medical authority, through privileging and representing the embodied experience of women's stories in live theatre performance.

Levelling hierarchies of knowledge to build dialogue

'Good theatre is the search for truths; it is often hard work. The process is not complete until we take our discoveries back into reality and apply them.' (Diamond, 1994: 36). The performances of *Daughters of the Revolution* were part of a search for those multiple truths, an acknowledgement of the divergent points of view that exist in all communities.

There are moments of change, seismic shifts in perception, where the invisible power structures are suddenly rendered visible (Shultzman, 1994: 140). The performances of *Daughters of the Revolution* were a powerful moment of public recognition for all the stories gathered from women and midwifery students. On each of the three nights, the audience engaged completely with the world created through the actors' embodiment of the physical and spoken language of the play. For a few hours, the audience became a community bound by the shared performance experience (Auslander, 1994: 126). The primacy of women's embodied knowledge represented on the stage, and the communal nature of the encounter allowed the people in the room to step out of their usual roles, and come to the discussion with a focused awareness of the multiple truths present there.

The theatre space exists outside the oppositional relationship of the usual statutory and institutional channels where discussions about the maternity services ordinarily take place. It enabled the development of the trust needed to ensure clear and effective communication and to explore concrete ways of working outside existing hierarchies of knowledge. We are all performing within the dominant social and cultural narrative but in this moment, in this space, that narrative was successfully disrupted.

Theatre of the Oppressed aspires to be inclusive and non-hierarchical in the creation and performance of theatrical pieces. I brought this practice to the facilitation of the post-show discussions. The expert panels in the post-show discussion were carefully balanced to represent both empirical and embodied knowledges. I reinforced this balance by explicitly and repeatedly recognising the value of all experiences in the room. By creating a safe and creative space for public and stakeholder engagement, *Daughters of the Revolution* provided a structure though which to share and reconcile the divergent perspectives of women, families, support staff, and health care professionals. The value of the experience and perspective of every person in the room was given equal weight. What was created was a model of how things could be. The performances created 'impossible encounters', bringing a range of people together that would not otherwise be in the same room. 'The hope behind the act lay in both its vivid present and its imagined future' (Heritage, 2004: 100).

The effectiveness of the performance could be best understood by the audience's response in the post-show discussions. Members of the audience spoke of being transported back to their own experiences of the maternity services and of the relief and affirmation they felt in seeing those experiences performed in a public space. By reclaiming the space for the counter-narrative of women's stories, embodied knowledge and the empirical knowledge of medical authority could have an equality of voice.

This levelling of knowledge hierarchies could be seen in the acceptance by health care professionals of the validity of the portrayal in *Daughters of the Revolution* and through that acceptance there was movement towards dialogue with women and families. This acceptance was not total, and there were many areas of negotiation that came up in the discussions. Issues arose, like how risk is constructed and how medical interventions in labour highlighted areas of direct conflict between medical, empirical and embodied knowledges. Balanced dialogue created openness to other perspectives, while the consultants and midwives spoke freely of the structural problems within the maternity services and their own frustrations with working within a flawed system.

There were many themes raised over the three nights, including: being listened to and feeling heard, access to information, continuity of care, feeling vulnerable and disempowered, and feeling that consultants had a disproportionate level of power compared to women in terms of deciding issues of care.

We found through the response to the post-show discussions that the culture of maternity services has a greater impact on the satisfaction of service users, and on staff morale and retention, than any other single factor. These observations reflect the conclusions of Health and Safety Executive (HSE) reports over the last ten years and the recommendations laid out in the National Maternity Strategy 2016–2026 (Ireland, Department of Health and Children, 2016).

The post-show discussions showed that listening and responding positively reduces negative outcomes, and even in the event of negative outcomes, the process of listening and responding itself reduces the potential for conflict and brings about solutions that satisfy the needs of all parties.

Theatre is not the revolution, it is a rehearsal for the revolution (Boal, 1979: 155), creating a model of what could be. Now, in the present we work to build relationships and share experiences and understandings that can begin to chart a course towards the future.

Daughters of the Revolution carried the potential to lead to better relationships and engage health care professionals and women in a shared experience of understanding, which in turn could lead to better communication and improved outcomes through modelling a process of parity of esteem, listening, and trust, firmly grounded in an equality of voice.

There were many concrete suggestions that came out of the post-show discussions:

- The funding allocated for maternity services should follow the individual women.
- Begin a programme of reproductive health education in all secondary schools run by midwives as part of the curriculum.
- Operate a system of mandatory open disclosure, including promoting a culture of listening and responding positively to a woman's and family concerns, as well as negative outcomes.

- Midwives to provide community education and resources to women and families along the continuum of reproductive health, from menstruation to menopause, to provide continuity of care throughout a woman's reproductive life.

Theatre performance is a fluid and dynamic practice that can represent and move between different social spheres: domestic, public, and hospital, and it can explore the interrelations between the different spheres through following the journey of one woman through the experience of maternity.

The use of theatre performance engages people in a creative experience. It invites a greater level of participation by the public by creating an entertaining and informal atmosphere. The theatre performance is designed to engage people emotionally and experientially in a shared event. Through the post-show discussions, problems could be framed and questions asked with parity of esteem and equality of voice.

The significance of *Daughters of the Revolution* lies in using creative theatre practice to open pathways to a dialogue that addresses and redresses the balance of power in the conversation on maternity in Ireland. Theatre creates a space outside the usual ways of acting and reacting; a space where empathy, dialogue, and trust can take root (Harris, 2016).

There is tremendous value to hospital professionals and service users in creating a shared space outside of the usual forms of interaction, taking part on a personal rather than purely professional level. The process of changing an organisational culture is incremental and time-intensive but can be done through working collaboratively with all stakeholders and by building personal relationships through respect, trust, and listening. Theatre brings individuals together to create a community through shared experience and the transformative nature of theatre unifies the multiple perspectives of individuals into the richer whole of collective experience.

13

DOCUMENTING EMPOWERMENT

Anne-Marie Green

Introduction

Documentary film has a long history of raising awareness of injustice. This chapter looks at how this creative form has been used to bring about change through informing and mobilising public opinion in Ireland to challenge Irish authorities on the crucial issue of accounting for maternal deaths. Through primary and secondary research, what I describe here is how an alternative space can be created to allow communities to discuss social issues, educate themselves and take action as part of a multi-pronged approach to campaigning. In an age of social media, documentaries can, more than ever, inform, empower and activate communities to campaign for change.

History of the form

The origins of the feature documentary film date back to *Nanook of the North* (1922) when Robert Flaherty charted the lives of the Inuit in Canada. Flaherty was fascinated by the survival skills of isolated people. He travelled to Samoa to film Polynesian villagers in *Moana* (1926) and to the Aran Islands for *Man of Aran* (1934), which documented the daily lives of islanders. This would later be called salvage ethnography – the recording of the practices and folklore of cultures threatened with extinction (Beattie, 2004). Flaherty's aim was to educate and inform his audience by showing a way of life that was fast disappearing. It created a legacy and preserved a past. Flaherty acknowledged the *tragedy* of the impending disappearance of a noble way of life but he did not comment on its *injustice*. He was merely showing life as it was.

This tradition of documenting life for current and future generations continued in the work of John Grierson who had originally coined the term 'documentary' during a review of Flaherty's work in the *New York Sun* (8 February 1926). Grierson, a Scot who served as first Commissioner on the National Film Board of Canada, created films that observed everyday life. In the 1920s and 1930s he made *Housing Problems*, dealing with slum eviction, and *Coal Face*, which depicted the working conditions of miners. Both films were powerful in their depiction of the actuality of working-class people's reality. This approach was also found in the work of Norwegian director Kristoffer Aamot in the 1940s who saw his work on contemporary Norway as 'a historical archive, documenting life which could be updated every twenty-five years.' (Brinch and Iversen, 2001).

The power of the medium to influence the viewing public through 'telling the truth' led it to be used for propaganda purposes. Leni Riefenstahl, often referred to as Hitler's favourite filmmaker, made *Triumph of the Will* about the 1934 Nazi rally in Nuremberg. It has been described as 'the best propaganda film ever' (Harding, 2003). Around the same time in the United States, President Franklin D. Roosevelt also employed the documentary form when introducing his post-Great Depression reforms known as the New Deal. He commissioned photographers and filmmakers to show the human and economic fallout of the 1929 financial collapse in the lives of thousands of impoverished Americans across the country in order to win over the taxpayers whose dollars would be used to finance the programme.

The birth of the social documentary

The social documentary with an implicit subjective commentary can be traced back before Flaherty's seminal work. In 1888 Jacob Riis, a police reporter, created a series of images called *The Other Half: How it Lives and Dies in New York*. His photographs 'remain classic documentary exposes of social inequities and division.' (Geiger, 2011). Riis, like Flaherty, was showing life as it was but his aim was different: 'Riis determined … to galvanize the public in a campaign to improve housing, health care, education, parks and the assimilation of the nation's growing immigrant population' (Roberts, 2015).

The social documentary therefore has a purpose other than to record and display. That purpose can be to raise awareness, to challenge, change or activate.

Raising awareness

The power of documentary film to inform a wide audience of a story with which they are mostly unfamiliar has become a mainstay of the form.

In recent years films such as *Gasland* (2010) and *Tapped* (2009) drew attention to the at best unethical activity on the part of large fossil fuel and water corporations.

A Turning Tide in the Life of Man (2015) by Loïc Jourdain follows the struggle of a fisherman living on Bo Finne Island off the northwest Irish coast to regain his ancestors' right to fish, which had been removed by the EU. A similar story was documented in Irish director Risteárd Ó Domhnaill's feature *Atlantic* (2016). His earlier film *The Pike* (2010) charted the Shell to Sea campaign against an onshore gas refinery in northwest Mayo. These Irish films look at contemporary contro-versial issues in Irish society involving political decisions at national and European level affecting local communities.

Some documentaries like *Gasland* grow out of personal experience. Former model Christy Turlington Burns who suffered a near fatal haemorrhage while giving birth to her first child directed *No Woman No Cry* (2010). It explores maternal mortality around the world and draws a comparison between the care she received with that provided to poor women in very low-income countries as well as in the United States where maternal mortality has been worryingly high and remains so (Gaskin, 2008). This emotional connection to the story is crucial to the impact of the documentary form where the filmmaker is shining a light on a little known or little understood social issue.

Challenge

Other films aim to challenge official 'truths', which Australian journalist and film-maker John Pilger described as 'often powerful illusions' (Bhatia, 2015). Pilger has exposed genocide in Cambodia, the manipulation of Latin America by the United States, the effect of economic sanctions on Iraq, and the betrayal of the East Timorese by the international community, as well as exposing the hidden political agendas of governments and regimes around the world. He urges his colleagues to question the official truths: 'Secretive power loathes journalists who do their job: push back screens, peer behind façades, lift rocks' (Pilger, 2004).

Pilger's films remind us to be sceptical of 'spin': the manipulation of facts. In the current era of 'fake news' challenging what is reported and published is more important than ever.

Change

Many documentary filmmakers see their role as independent truth tellers. They record events as they happen with the aim of forcing those whom their work regards as 'guilty' to publicly concede their lies. For others, they see their work as having the power to alter current practice and ameliorate the lives of those affected in the future.

In films such as *Supersize Me* (2004) and *Wal-Mart: The High Cost of Low Price* (2005) the targets are the corporations who the filmmakers believe contribute to a social injustice. In the former, Morgan Spurlock ate nothing but McDonald's fast food for 30 days to draw attention to obesity in the United States. In the latter, Robert Greenwald exposes the poor working conditions and business practices of the supermarket corporation. Michael Moore's work engages with many contem-porary issues in American society including the gun lobby, the health insurance industry and globalisation. His examination of the Bush administration's invasion of Iraq and Afghanistan made *Fahrenheit 9/11* the most commercially successful documentary ever made, grossing nearly 120 million US dollars (thelostboy, 2011).

Such films have multiple roles. They raise awareness among citizens, shame the company or organisation into changing their practices and, failing that, pressurise governments to outlaw unacceptable practices.

Activate

> With organization you have the aid of your fellow man. Without organi-zation you are a lone individual without influence and without recognition of any kind.
>
> *John L. Lewis, President, United Mine Workers of America, 1920–1960*

John L. Lewis may have been talking about the trade union movement but his words apply to any group of people who commit to stand together in defence or in pursuit of human rights. The power of the collective can be tremendous but it first needs to be galvanised.

Films that aim to *activate* a group of people, a 'public', need to engage at a deeper level with their audience (Aufderheide, 2007: 5). They need to be part of a wider movement that can harness audience reaction and focus it on action. They are implicitly political.

David Guggenheim's film *An Inconvenient Truth* (2006), which follows former USA presidential candidate Al Gore's campaign to raise public awareness of the dangers of global warming, proved a rallying cry. The climate change movement now operates at many levels:

1   Individual – recycling, domestic energy efficiency
2   Community – grassroots movements developing energy resilience within local communities
3   Government – financial support for fuel-saving technology
4   Political – Green Party, environment ministries
5   Global – International Panel on Climate Change, emissions agreements, carbon trading.

The environmental movement has had a transformative effect on people's behaviour: at grassroots level people feel they have a responsibility and the power to make a contribution to change. 'When people and communities are armed with information, imagination, and the ability to engage with one another, we can change public will, our actions, and impacts.' (Friedenwald-Fishman, 2011).

Case study

The powerful documentary *It's a Girl* (2012) tackles the issue of gendercide, the systematic killing of members of a specific sex. The film looks at female infanticide, primarily in India and China where, in certain provinces, the ratio of very young men to very young women runs as high as 140 to 100. *It's a Girl* helps to piece together what has happened to the 200 million girls the UN estimates are missing worldwide.

The documentary is an inspiring example of how art can become part of a wider call to action. The website www.itsagirlmovie.com shows a trailer and a synopsis, a list of screenings and a blog. It facilitates the publicising through traditional and online media of the documentary by including a downloadable press kit. It provides an educational version of the documentary for use in schools and libraries. Cinema releases for documentaries are limited but by allowing communities to host a screening outside the cinema circuit the documentary makers are using the community to increase viewership.

Under its *Take Action* tab, it has a number of options to allow viewers to channel their emotional response to the film through concrete action that is easy to carry out:

- Two step ready-to-click connection to pre-existing petitions to end female genocide in India and China
- Donate to charities that support Indian and Chinese NGOs working to combat gendercide
- Encouraging sharing through the *Invite A Friend* tab
- Social media sharing facilitated through Facebook, Twitter and Tumblr
- Share tab for the campaign's manifesto
- Downloadable *Discussion + Action Guide* to help start a group discussion after viewing the film.

This last option allows working at a very deep community level. Through facilitating discussion after the showing of the documentary, local communities explore their thoughts and emotions provoked by the film and these forums can stimulate new ways of working to bring about change that the main campaign had not thought of.

The *It's a Girl* campaign is an example of a well-thought-through, multifaceted advocacy programme that uses the documentary to spearhead this deeper engagement. This type of approach is broadly described as 'intelligence work' in Kahana: 'An audience comes to understand itself as an agent of change when it figures out how to generalize from the case on screen to other situations and cases.' (Kahana, 2008).

Political mimesis

The potential of film to influence and activate viewers' behaviour is what Gaines (1999) calls 'political mimesis'. Tay (2006) gives the example of Irish bus driver Tom Hyland from Ballyfermot in Dublin who felt compelled to work for Timorese independence after viewing '*Cold Blood: The Massacre of East Timor*'. The documentary showed footage of the massacre in the cemetery of Santa Cruz where Indonesian troops and police opened fire on the East Timorese.

Despite being unaware of the struggle for independence in East Timor, the documentary had such a profound effect on Hyland that he got involved in activism immediately. He set up the East Timor Ireland Solidarity Campaign and spent years working tirelessly to put the small country on the political agenda. He subsequently moved to what is now called Timor Leste where he held a government post.

Picking Up the Threads

The origin of the making of the documentary, *Picking Up the Threads,* shares similar objectives and in its making evolved as a more clearly defined activist project. It was initially meant to record the creation of a commemorative quilt by midwives, midwifery students and birth activists to express their solidarity with young healthy mothers dying in, or shortly after, childbirth in Ireland (see Chapter 15). The quilt itself focused on eight women for whom inquests had been held, as described in Chapter 14. The original intention for the film, following on from the inquests, was to screen it at midwifery conferences and to student midwives. Around the same time, an independent Irish deputy, Teachta Dála (TD) and activist, Clare Daly, who had become involved in the fight for an earlier inquest, introduced a private member's bill into the Irish Parliament to allow for mandatory inquests after all maternal deaths. This became an important focus for the documentary.

As filming progressed, its scope grew to include interviews with partners of women who had died, and this changed the target audience. The film was now aiming for the general public, whose support for political change could be harnessed. The exhibition, which included the quilt, the documentary, portraits of each of the women by Clare-based artist Martina Hynan (Chapter 14) and later a video installation by student artist Laura Fitzpatrick, began to tour the country. The campaign was called the Elephant Collective (see Chapter 14). Contacts were made with local individuals or groups, already working within the field of birthing and improvements to maternity care, who were willing to host the exhibition.

Each showing of the film has been followed by an open floor debate. Members of the Elephant Collective take questions and comments and clarify and add updates to the work done by the campaign. The partners of women who have died are frequently in attendance. Their contribution is invaluable, both in the documentary and in person, in making all too real the issue of maternal death. Their testimony underlines the widespread devastation caused by a maternal death. Partners are left to care perhaps for a new-born as well as for other children, mourn their loss, and commonly fight a long and very lonely battle to gain the inquest and to find out what happened. At each exhibition, we have made a comments book available with the option to leave a contact email address. This has proven a useful resource for keeping viewers involved in the campaign.

Response to the documentary

A brief questionnaire survey, carried out among viewers of *Picking Up the Threads* in 2016, explored responses to the film and ways in which people felt they would be willing to assist the campaign. More than 100 people who left email addresses in our comments book were contacted to ask them ten questions using a simple online Survey Monkey tool.

There were responses from 21 of those contacted. The first question was how people had heard of the film. An equal number – 20 per cent – had heard through social media or by reading a poster. Less than 7 per cent had heard through traditional media – newspapers or radio. More than 50 per cent had heard through family or friends. This might suggest people were coming just to accompany friends or family. Indeed the second question 'What is your connection to the film?' revealed that a quarter of respondents said their relative or friend was involved in making the film or in the Elephant Collective. But 40 per cent said they were involved in activism. This would suggest that making contact with other activist groups could be a way of spreading word of the campaign.

When asked 'What new information did you learn from watching the documentary?' there was a range of responses. The scale of the problem, the number of maternal deaths and the lack of mandatory inquests featured strongly.

> *That there is no automatic inquest following a maternal death. That it is the hospital itself that files an initial report into the death.*

> *The number of avoidable deaths (having only been aware of some of them), and the unconscionable response of the hospitals concerned to the bereaved families.*

The effect on the partners also had a strong impact.

> *How the day to day living for widowers is after the maternal death. How drawn out the process of obtaining an inquest is.*

> *…the horrendous journey by partners looking for answers, for accountability, and how little info & support there is for them.*

All respondents agreed with the campaign's core purpose, to seek mandatory inquests in cases of maternal death. They saw three important outcomes:

- To help partners grieve
  All maternal deaths must be investigated to give answers to family members.
  In order to properly grieve and come to terms with such tragic loss it is important to know what happened, and why.

- Accountability

If a woman dies in childbirth, that's unacceptable in this country, so there must be speedy mandatory inquests, holding all relevant parties accountable.

- Improvement to services

When things go wrong, the causal factors must be identified and practice changed!

Of course all cases should be investigated, both for the sake of the families and for the medical profession so that they can learn but also so that we can all learn and work towards avoiding them in the future.

Translating response into action

Eliciting an empathetic response through a documentary on a social issue is just the first step to bringing about change. The next is to facilitate viewers to go further and take concrete action. The final questions in the survey deal with what kind of action viewers of the film would be prepared to take to help achieve the aims of the campaign.

Again, traditional media did not score highly, with fewer than one in five respondents saying they would write to a newspaper. On the other hand nearly 60 per cent said they would spread the word of the Elephant Collective via social media.

An equal percentage, 61.9 per cent, of people said they would be prepared to either contact their local political representatives on the issue and/or join a local group sharing the aims of the Elephant Collective campaign.

More than 70 per cent said they would send a pre-written letter to politicians and media organisations.

Over three-quarters of respondents said they would fill in a petition.

These responses indicate that, as with the *It's a Girl* campaign, the key to turning response into action is making it relatively simple for viewers to act.

When asked what actions viewers *had* taken, almost two-thirds (61.1 per cent) had spread the word via social media.

The final question in the survey called for suggestions for further action that the Elephant Collective could undertake.

…organise a dedicated campaign on fb (Facebook) until mandatory inquests are achieved.

Keep showing the documentary, partner with small community groups for viewings.

Attending any events. Speaking venues. Social media petitions and campaigns […] join women's groups discussions.

Get the word out to all women's groups, men's groups like the Men's Sheds etc,

Facebook posts, regular talks etc.

As evidenced by the responses, viewers see social media as a powerful tool to help spread news and information about the campaign. However, many of the respondents wanted to see the documentary and exhibition shown to a wider public, including the medical profession and women's and men's groups. This last suggestion echoes a call by the partners of the women remembered in the documentary for men to become involved in the campaign, and to educate themselves on the issues so that they can better protect wives and partners.

Conclusion

We can see that the documentary has multiple purposes in dealing with social issues. Human rights films serve to inform and educate viewers about stories that are often hidden. They give voice to victims. As part of a multi-stranded campaign, especially through social media, they can communicate with a wider audience and can activate communities by involving them in screening and distribution. The documentary can leverage public outrage to force political awareness and ultimately bring about legal change. It can have that quality of political mimesis where to act becomes vital to the person who is made aware of deep injustice.

Picking Up the Threads has had the effect of sensitising viewers to the individual tragedy that lies behind the news headlines. It introduces the audience to the women who died, not as statistics but as mothers, partners, daughters, sisters. Their partners' pain is tangible. Yet they are ordinary people who have lived through extraordinary tragedy. By bringing their humanity to the fore the documentary underlines the fact that it could happen to anyone.

At a deeper level, the documentary can have a profound and more long-term effect on how people behave. In her exploration of the work of a group of film-makers documenting human rights abuses in Mexico, Hinegardner (2009) sums it up. For these filmmakers who have no hope of having the legal and political system respond to their work she says, 'the goal of making films is not to change laws but to create a new culture of politics [in Mexico] ... through organizing a community in which abuse[s] are not tolerated'.

Picking Up the Threads, through informing women and men of what has happened and continues to happen in Irish maternity care, will, it is hoped, not only lead to mandatory inquests for all maternal deaths, but challenge the maternity services to greatly improve their care and the accountability for their care. Just as importantly is the creation of an informed and empowered community that finds its voice and uses it to combat all forms of social injustice.

14

HIDDEN IN PLAIN SIGHT

Mapping the erasure of the maternal body from visual culture

Martina Hynan

Background

> Hidden in Plain Sight: be unnoticeable, by staying visible in a setting that masks presence.
>
> *(yourdictionary, 2017)*

> ...the struggle, over women's access to and control over their reproduction is not a matter of medical and legal rights alone. It is also a matter of cultural politics that can engage with ...ways that contest the medical, political and media images and practices through which these are currently framed.
>
> *Betterton (1996: 128)*

An obstetrically led way of seeing the birthing body has developed since the eighteenth century that has affected both medical professionals' vision of childbirth and that of the birthing woman. The obstetric gaze refers to specific ways that man-midwives saw the birthing body primarily from a surgical interventionist perspective that led to a new way of seeing and assisting women in childbirth. The experience of childbirth is effectively hidden in plain sight, the plain sight of the obstetric gaze that is encouraged within our maternity systems. The evolution of this way of seeing childbirth has relied heavily on the collaboration between art and medicine to create a fragmented, compartmentalised, mechanistic vision of the birthing body that concurrently erases the experience of childbirth itself.

The maternal body is therefore a contested site medically, socially, culturally and politically, and this also includes maternal deaths. A need to understand how maternal deaths are dealt with in Ireland led to a national campaign that has made these tragic deaths visible (see Chapter 15).

In 2014, along with fellow members of Clare Birth Choice, a birth activist group, I knitted panels for inclusion in a quilt being made to commemorate the eight women who died between 2007 and 2013 in the Irish maternity services and whose families struggled to secure inquests into these sudden and tragically unexpected deaths. The inquest verdicts made their deaths visible, which ultimately led to the creation of the multimedia art exhibition *Picking Up the Threads: Remaking the Fabric of Care*.

However, concrete change within the existing maternity system can only happen when women's experiences of childbirth are seen from a new perspective. Unless and until this happens, childbirth will remain hidden in plain sight.

A brief overview of the history of the obstetric gaze

A direct line of vision can be drawn from the historical eighteenth-century physician attending women in labour, to the modern incarnation of the consultant obstetrician at the top of the professional hierarchy. This line, grounded in unequal relations of power, highlights the consistently patriarchal way of seeing the birthing body.

Two of the earliest man-midwives who used anatomical illustrations to promote their work were William Smellie (1697–1763) and William Hunter (1718–1783). Smellie and Hunter drew on the skills of landscape painter turned medical artist, Jan Van Rymsdyk, (c.1730–1788/89) who illustrated the books that became known as atlases for both William Smellie and William Hunter. Van Rymsdyk's detailed works demonstrate his skill as an artist but also reveal Smellie and Hunter's preferred interpretation of the female body. Both the baby and the forceps are described in great detail, and the intensity of the drawing is testament to Van Rymsdyk's ability to look at the subject in close-up; however, the specific aspects of the woman's body and the lack of reference to her limbs or skin concentrate the viewer's eye on the inter-relationship between the forceps and the baby. The virtual invisibility of the mother in this process suggests that her involvement in birth is minimal and passive. This concept of women's passivity in the medical sphere has been much written about, concentrating on the social impact of passivity from a gendered perspective (Fissell, 2004; Jordanova, 1989; Murphy-Lawless, 1988, 1998; Schiebinger, 1993).

Hunter considered Van Rymsdyk's illustrations to be a merely personal vision of the *gravid uterus* and therefore felt no compulsion to acknowledge him in the publication of his atlas in 1774. However, Massey (2005: 83) suggests that Van Rymsdyk 'helped invent the visual language on which Hunter's atlas depends', moreover, the images 'were clearly intended to signify Hunter's notion of pure objectivity'. This obstetric gaze has consistently relied on artistic aesthetics to bolster its view of the birthing body (Massey, 2005; Kemp, 1992; Korsmeyer, 2004) and to reinforce its claim to objectivity. Their interventionist vision of a fragmented body is based on their scientific reading of the body that subordinates the experience of the pregnant woman to the authority of the medical professional.

Nineteenth-century aesthetic theorisations of the body extended these meanings in a fluid interchange between masculinist artistic and medical approaches to seeing the body. Here in Ireland, the work of Dr John Woodroffe (1781–1859), surgeon and midwifery lecturer who taught anatomical drawing to artists at the Royal Dublin Society in the 1840s (Turpin, 1986), provides one example of this crossover. The travelling anatomical museum, owned by Dr Joseph Kahn, provides a second. This latter was exhibited at the Rotunda Rooms, Dublin, in 1853. Kahn's museum contained the by then traditional wax models of women's pregnant bodies, including an anatomical Venus (Kahn, 1853).

The effective deletion of the mother's body from a scientific model of birth from these earlier periods has become a standard vision of birth in contemporary visual culture whereby reproductive medicine is taught. This is a history that has prioritised the male creative interpretation of the inner working of the birthing body, actively denying women's participation in the process of birth.

Feminist interventions: An/other way of seeing the birthing body

From the 1960s, an emerging feminist discourse on the body, sexuality and gender included explorations of how the birthing body had come to be seen and not seen (Rich, 1976). Childbirth features in the work of many women artists during this era and their work was very challenging to audiences. For example, Monica Sjoo's painting *God Giving Birth* (1968) was considered blasphemous when first exhibited. In fact it was based on Sjoo's memories of the home birth of her second child in 1961. This experience of the power of her birthing body changed Sjoo irrevocably and led her to question the patriarchal view of women's bodies (Sjoo, 1973). Others too were questioning how women's birthing bodies were seen and how they could be seen (Kelly, 1983; Broude and Garrard, 1996).

The artist Judy Chicago examined the history of birth imagery in the canon of Western art and was 'dismayed' how few images there were (Chicago, 1985). She addressed this 'puzzling omission' in *The Birth Project*, designing multiple images on the subject of birth and employing needle workers from the United States, Canada and New Zealand to create the art pieces. It was exhibited over 100 times in the 1980s and the works are currently displayed in various museums and are frequently used as part of university curricula. Chicago (cited in Sackler, 2002: 68) asserts that to see the vulva in labour is to be 'confronted with sheer female power'.

At the same time that *The Birth Project* was raising questions about the power of the birthing body in society, Ireland was facing many questions about women's birthing bodies from a different perspective. In 1984, there were two very high-profile cases that dominated the media and public imagination. On 31 January 1984, Ann Lovett, a 15-year-old girl, died shortly after giving birth alone in a Marian grotto in Granard, Co. Longford (Maguire, 2001). Her death came just four months after the Eighth Amendment of the Constitution Act (1983) which amended Article 40.3.3 of the constitution, to enshrine that the state 'acknowledge[s] the right to life of the unborn and, with due regard to the equal right to life of the mother' (Eighth Amendment of the Constitution Act, 1983).

In July 1984, artist Pauline Cummins completed the mural *Celebration* for the National Maternity Hospital, Dublin as part of the Irish Exhibition of Living Art, just six months after Ann's death. The mural was erased within a month of its completion without consulting Cummins.

Twenty-one years later, during an interview with art historian Katy Deepwell, Cummins reflected on her feelings about her work being destroyed without any consultation: 'I was upset when they painted the mural out, but I wasn't completely surprised. I don't like saying they weren't ready for it, but it obviously was too early' (Pauline Cummins cited in Deepwell, 2005: 39).

Cummins's desire to celebrate birth came at a particularly fraught time. The tragedy of Ann Lovett's death at the end of January was followed by what became known as the Kerry Babies Case (McCafferty, 1985; Maguire, 2001; Inglis, 2003). Between April and October 1984, the media focused relentlessly on the case of Joanne Hayes who was charged with infanticide when the body of a new-born baby was found brutally murdered on a beach in Caherciveen, Co. Kerry. Despite the fact that forensic evidence proved that neither Hayes nor her partner could be the parents of the dead baby, the Gardaí (the Irish police) continued to insist that she was in fact the mother. Hayes had given birth alone in a field on the family farm shortly before her arrest in April. The baby had died at birth and she had buried him in the field. It was suggested that if she were capable of this act then she was also capable of infanticide.

When Cummins created her mural at the National Maternity Hospital in July 1984, the case of the Kerry Babies was dominating the media. For the mural, Cummins decided to draw on a painting made during her second pregnancy when she sought to reclaim history painting and looked at 'heroic paintings of battle scenes, but it [the painting] celebrates birth instead' (Pauline Cummins cited in Deepwell, 2005: 39).

However, when Cummins showed the same image as a painting in an art gallery, she 'felt that the audience didn't know what I was talking about' (Deepwell, 2005: 39) with the audience apparently unable to engage with the image. Cummins then approached the maternity hospital with the idea of creating a mural based on the painting, hoping that in the hospital setting, 'people would understand the experience' of childbirth as a time of celebration (ibid.).

This experience of erasure forced Cummins to reconsider her working methodology. Later in 1984, she created her slide-text art piece, *Nine Months and After*. Reflecting on this work, Cummins said she was 'trying to bridge the gap between the experience of childbirth and motherhood, a theme often excluded from the art world because those experiences were not acceptable material at the time in Ireland' (ibid.).

Cummins returned to the National Maternity Hospital in 1994, together with artist Louise Walsh, to create an installation piece called *Sounding the Depths*, which was part of the hospital's centenary celebrations (Irvine, 1992).

During this exhibition another artist, Kate Malone, in a piece called *Viewer* placed photographs in light-boxes in different locations around the hospital. The nursing manager of the fetal assessment unit asked Kate to remove the image of a pregnant woman's torso and replace it with the image of an ultrasound. This request was made on behalf of the women attending the unit. As the exhibition curator Grehan (2007: 57) notes, this 'suggests that the expectant women were more comfortable with the images of the interior of their womb than the exterior of their abdomen'.

This is an emphatic example of the established authority of the obstetric gaze. While Kate's work was not erased, in the way that Pauline's had been ten years earlier, it was nonetheless changed in such a way that it presented an acceptable mode of seeing childbirth which reinforced the obstetric vision of the birthing body and denied an alternative vision of the pregnant body from being seen within the maternity institutional setting.

Portraits as part of *Picking up the Threads: Remaking the Fabric of Care*

Maternal identity in Ireland continues in its struggle to be visible on many levels (Murphy-Lawless, 1988; Betterton, 1996, Murphy-Lawless, 1998; Deepwell, 2005; Pollock, 2009; Tyler and Baraitser, 2013). In the context of the multimedia exhibition, *Picking Up the Threads: Remaking the Fabric of Care*, it seemed to me that portraits of the eight women being commemorated should be seen alongside the quilt made up from over 100 individual contributions (Photograph 14.1). For me, the portraits are a visible reminder of an uneasy truth in our society that women die in our maternity services as a result of errors in that system. The maternal gaze of the women in these portraits is intended to bring the viewer up against the power of the gaze, the obstetric and the maternal, and our need to engage with and challenge the parameters of both.

Their enduring maternal gaze tells another story of the women who have been historically hidden in plain sight. I created the portraits in an attempt to make this patriarchal history of birth more visible. The experience of women artists in Ireland and the experience of Irish women giving birth are linked by their common assertion of needing to be heard in the national dialogue against the evolution of a privileged obstetric gaze. The latter persistently draws heavily on aesthetic theorisations of the birthing body, echoing the dominance of the male gaze in visual culture itself. It was important to me that these portraits supported our desire to commemorate women and highlight the maternal gaze of the women being remembered.

Images of seven of the eight women were sourced from the public domain, from newspaper articles posted online where I found small photographs embedded in the articles with details about the inquest findings. There were none of Jennifer Crean. However, when contacted and asked for an image as part of this project, Jennifer's husband Francis very kindly sent a photograph that I then used to create a portrait of Jennifer. The names of all the women and their dates of death are listed beneath the photograph of the portraits accompanying this chapter (Photograph 14.2).

These eight women had been united in death and their families were united in their struggles to navigate a path through the coronial system to secure inquests. I decided that I would unite them in scale and palette as well. The portraits are A1 in size, which means their faces are larger than life-size.

I was aware that the families and children of the women would see the portraits and this prompted me to retain a fundamentally realistic style of painting. However, I did modify and adjust the images moderately so that when the paintings are hung the eyes of the women are at the same level. I also accentuated the eyes of the women to draw attention to their gaze in the space. It was important to me that not only would people see a representation of the women being commemorated but that the way they were painted would emphasise their maternal gaze. Finally, I decided to use the same colour and tonal range for each painting, creating another level of visual connection.

Working across the portraits simultaneously allowed me to develop an inter-relationship with each image. As I painted, I read and re-read the circumstances of each woman's death. Staring into the images of these faces and knowing how they died and that they had left behind partners, and in many cases children, reinforced my decision to retain a strong representational element to the portraits with a gentle emphasis on the eyes of each woman.

Exhibiting: Curatorial decisions

We have consciously sought venues that are well known locally, nationally and internationally as well as being welcoming to community groups.

To date the exhibition has been shown in nine venues. When it was initially launched in November 2015, at the Dublin Institute of Technology, the exhibition consisted of: the knitted quilt, with a border of 400 elephants, designed and knitted by Mary Smyth and Ann Maxwell (Photograph 14.3), representing how elephants surround the cow as she is giving birth to protect her; seven of the eight portraits; an embroidered, framed panel with the eight women's names; and a trailer for Anne-Marie Green's documentary (see Chapter 13). Both song and poetry accom-panied this first showing, performed by drama students from the Dublin Institute of Technology, directed by Mary Moynihan. There was also a box heaped high with wool. Visitors to the exhibition were invited to contribute a few stitches to an ongoing spontaneous expression of support, and the box with its ever-lengthening piece has travelled with the exhibition. The exhibition currently includes the above, all eight portraits, the completed documentary, and also a short film by artist Laura Fitzpatrick with an accompanying book. Her work is called *Silent Killer*. This last joined the exhibition in September 2016 when it was shown alongside a screening of the full documentary at the Wexford Film Festival. We also have work from local knitting groups who have created pieces in response to seeing the exhibition and which now travel with it. These were coordinated by one of the skilled knitters in the Elephant Collective, Doreen Fitzmaurice, who invited local craft groups in Donegal, Clare, and Galway to come in for sessions during the exhibition's runs to discuss the problems besetting our maternity services and to reflect on the tragedy of the women's deaths.

We chose venues that have cultural and social integrity which also retain strong connections within their local communities, making them ideal settings for groups to spend time with the exhibition. Other venues offered audiences a different way of engaging with the work. For example, when we exhibited at the Institute for Lifecourse and Society, National University of Ireland, Galway, we hosted a panel discussion that included an international human rights lawyer, a midwifery professor, a practising midwife, a county councillor, and a solicitor working with women to secure their rights in childbirth. In Ormston House, in Limerick, on International Women's Day 2017, a group of local women performed a short play they had written. In Wexford, again coordinated by Doreen Fitzmaurice and picking up the theme of the quilt's elephant border, a local community development group made small ceramic elephants and collected 500 postcards with images of the quilt, signed by members of the public, asking for the legislation to be passed, and they sent these to the Minister for Justice in support of the legislative campaign seeking mandatory inquests for all maternal deaths in Ireland (see Chapter 15). Wherever it has gone, the exhibition has received local and national press, television and radio coverage; two of the widowers, Michael Kivlehan and Sean Rowlette, have given extensive interviews about their experiences, and the depth of their loss.

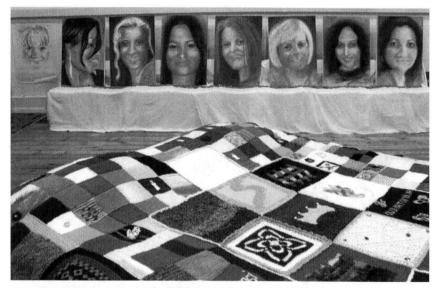

PHOTOGRAPH 14.1 Launch of exhibition, *Picking up the Threads: Remaking the Fabric of Care*, Dublin Institute of Technology, November 2015. (Photograph by Theo Hynan-Ratcliffe)

The exhibition will continue to embody a forceful grassroots statement from across Ireland of the need for radical change in our maternity services.

Conclusion

Our maternity services are dominated by the obstetric gaze that permeates our medical, social and political understanding of the experience of childbirth. The maternal gaze is marginalised and rendered invisible, shrouded in the miasma of a patriarchal system that systematically controls every aspect of the experience of giving birth.

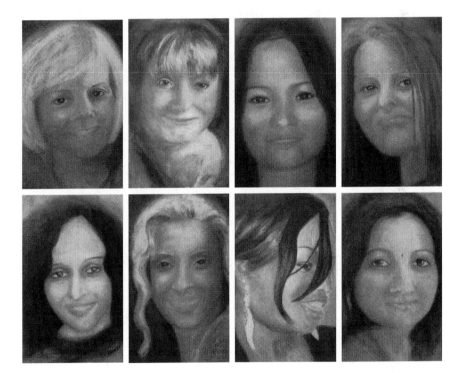

PHOTOGRAPH 14.2 Portraits of eight women whose inquests revealed their deaths were caused by medical misadventure. L to R: Evelyn Flanagan died 19 October 2007, Jennifer Crean died 10 February 2009, Nora Hyland died 13 February 2012, Sally Rowlette died 5 February 2013, Dhara Kivlehan died 28 September 2010, Tania McCabe died 9 March 2007, Bimbo Onanuga died 4 March 2010, Savita Halappanavar died 28 October 2012. (Photographs by Theo Hynan-Ratcliffe)

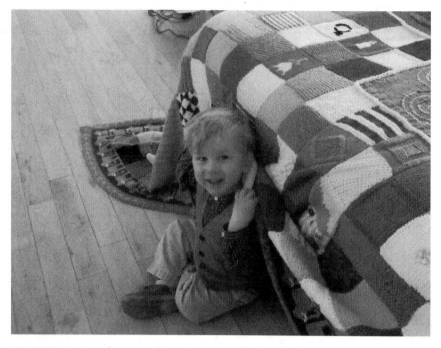

PHOTOGRAPH 14.3 A young visitor interacts with the Elephant Border, *Picking Up the Threads* Exhibition, Ennistymon Courthouse Gallery, September, 2016. (Photograph by Theo Hynan-Ratcliffe)

The commemorative portraits, which are just one element of the evolving multimedia exhibition, draw attention to the absent presence of eight specific women who died as a result of mistakes made during their care in the Irish maternity services. In the portraits they return the viewers' gaze in a steadfast attempt to highlight not only their plight and that of others but also to challenge the viewer to find other ways of seeing the birthing body.

Working with the multimedia exhibition has highlighted the need for comprehensive change in our maternity system, but it also has taught me the vital importance of perception and visual culture to the process. Art and birth are integrally linked, both personally and politically. We must restore a female creative vision to a maternity system that has been overly influenced by a male perspective, allowing the potential of individuality, art and language to return back to the heart of a mother's birth experience to heal maternity through the power of the maternal.

15

RESPONDING TO THE TRAGEDY OF MATERNAL DEATH

A collective challenges the state

Jo Murphy-Lawless

Introduction: A woman's death and its impact

For the past eleven years, I have been privileged to teach sociology to undergraduate pre-registration midwives in Trinity College Dublin. Their four-year degree comprises academic, theoretical and practical work on the physiology, psychology and sociology of pregnancy and birth, emphasising the contexts of women's lives as pregnant and new mothers. They also carry out three clinical placements in each of their first three years before commencing a 26-week internship in their fourth year. These clinical placements are in two of the three stand-alone maternity hospitals in Dublin, either the Rotunda or the Coombe; hospitals with a history stretching back 270 years.

Sadly, as elsewhere, maternity services in Ireland are broken, albeit against a background of a far more absolutist medical profession than in the UK. In 2008, the Health Services Executive (HSE), an arms' length body running the Irish health services on behalf of the Department of Health and Children, commissioned the international accountancy group KPMG to carry out a detailed review of maternity services in the greater Dublin area. The three maternity hospitals: the Coombe, the Rotunda and the National Maternity Hospital accounted for 40 per cent of all births in Ireland, each managing at least 8,000 births per annum. Since 2008, numbers per hospital on occasion have risen to well over 9,000 per annum. Against these numbers, KPMG recorded a total staff shortage of 296 clinicians among the three hospitals, including 221 midwives (KPMG, 2008: 6–7).

By 2008, Ireland was already caught up in the international economic collapse which was to see Irish Gross National Product (GNP) fall by 13 per cent between then and 2010 as the country entered deep recession. Like the UK and other EU countries, Ireland subjected its public services to draconian cutbacks while ordinary citizens faced punitive wage cuts, income tax rises and job losses to pay the debts of commercial banking institutions, which had been 'no more than casinos' (O'Toole, 2010: 7) for players in a globalised economy. This zombie global 'growth' regime had created still more insecurity internationally, with the circumstances of ordinary people's lives markedly declining along with their health (Marmot, 2016). Nonetheless, the Irish state was fully signed up to protecting what Lazzarato (2009) terms the 'enterprise society' and with it the neoliberal social policy with its market orientation, which eviscerates public services. Under this regime, our maternity services were not going to change for the better in the foreseeable future.

The multiple impacts of these complex conditions have meant that the students' clinical placements are frequently extremely stressful. Any individual woman's circumstances in pregnancy, labour and after birth can present unpredictable challenges where our students are suddenly called on to be there with the whole of their ethical selves, say, when a baby is unexpectedly still-born. However, the brokenness of our maternity services demands far more of them on a daily basis. The scope of care for women in this most intimate and vulnerable period has been ruthlessly cut away by a system suffering severe under-staffing and lack of resources, a system which suffers from chronic inadequate management, which is poorly acquainted with current and emerging evidence, and which remains stuck in its traditional patriarchal mode, with deeply unequal relations of power pressing down on women and students alike.

Maternity hospitals and units form one part of a health service for which the state claims overall responsibility in maintaining the national good and well-being. A Foucauldian perspective on the state might also point out that within its task of seeing to that good (and thus preserving its own legitimacy), it takes on what in older political language was termed a task of 'policing': the state exerts a 'permanent intervention' in 'social processes' (Foucault, 2002: 414–15). It does so through an accretion of myriad structures, institutions, and regulations, all exercising different forms of power which are 'superimposed', which 'cross over, limit and in some cases annul, in others reinforce' existing forms of power. Thus, although vast networks of 'power relations' involving everyday life have been progressively 'rationalized, and centralized … under the auspices of state institutions' insofar as 'all other forms of power relations must refer to it [the state]' (Foucault, 2002: 345), they are uneven in effect. Therefore they are also always open to possibilities of contestation, to a 'strategy of struggle' (ibid.: 347), and to being overturned in order to redress inequalities of power, even at the worst of times, such as those following the 2008 collapse.

My task is to help students to see, to make sense of, to be able to analyse these conditions of practice where they work, to understand how relations of power operate, and to develop the confidence, understanding, and skills to confront poor practice. For example, why is it that the Irish state has been prepared to license, more or less unquestioningly, the continuing hierarchy of professional obstetric power in the running of its maternity services, and by so doing permit the subordination of the voices and experiences of women and of midwives, whereas elsewhere in its operations, the notion of equality has long since been established as a legal good? In the terms of Jacques Rancière (2007), this broken space of the maternity services opens up the potential to develop a collective dissensus that confronts 'a policing order'.

On the 21 March 2010, my then third-year students returned to college from a six-week placement. They had a morning seminar with me. At once, it was evident that something was badly wrong: they were visibly upset, spirits rock bottom:

> 'What is it' I asked them, 'what's happened?'
> 'Jo, did no one tell you about the Nigerian woman who died?'
> 'No, no one has said a word to me.'

We spent the remainder of our time discussing their understanding of how on the 4 March, Bimbo Onanuga, a pregnant Nigerian, registered as an asylum-seeker, had come to die. I returned home that night to what was the beginning of a project which would challenge current institutional and state rationality, not that I could possibly have recognised that at the outset. Initially, the crucial matter was that my students were distressed about the events leading up to Bimbo's death. Senior hospital management fell back on explanations which had a sort of logic, a making sense of a catastrophe, but which also placed them outside events, closing off the complexity of multiple truths while asserting their own account.

The students, none of whom were immediately involved in the care of the dying woman, were unable to shed the sense that local hospital responses were insufficient in the face of this catastrophe; they were troubled by the detail, for example of a hospital bed not able to fit beyond the door to get to a nearby operating theatre with a by then critically ill woman. Surely there must be an institutional responsibility about a basic facet of care before the fact, not after it.

Theirs was the weight of an ethical sensibility, what Zygmunt Bauman terms a 'moral proximity' (1993: 217) which could not be eclipsed despite the determinism of schedules, of protocols and regulations, of all the machinery of our contemporary way of doing things, which seeks to normalise what cannot and should not be made normal. My question to myself that night was what must be my response, what must I do for my students to support them in their insupportable burden of an alternative possibility, of a woman sent to her death through negligence?

Obstetrics and its truth

Obstetrics won its ground as a science worthy of respect largely on its claims that it could rescue women from death. In the seventeenth, eighteenth and nineteenth centuries, accounts like the following of a woman dying from puerperal fever were the staple of obstetric chronicles and they laid a claim to a particular truth:

No. 12 28 years of age, second pregnancy, unmarried, caught cold in a railway train coming up from County Meath, was lying in a lodging house for a week ... Peritoneal symptoms set in immediately after delivery, between which and distress of mind she sank on the fourth day.

(Johnston 1869: 108)

This passage, from the clinical records of George Johnston, Master of the Rotunda Hospital from 1868 to 1875, has haunted me from the first moment I encountered it. There is the all too brief glimpse of a woman, without a name, who flees to Dublin in post-Famine years when unmarried women giving birth also bore an increasingly heavy burden of stigma.

We can try to see her: that railway carriage, searching out the boarding house until she senses she is in labour, dragging herself to the Rotunda, which was the only public facility of the period where unmarried women could go to give birth and leave again (unlike the workhouses).

Johnston uses this account as part of his analysis on why the use of forceps is beneficial for unmarried women in particular because they suffer greatly from what he termed 'remorse and fretting' about their pregnant unmarried state, and thus must be got through labour as quickly as possible. He took to applying the forceps on women who were as little as two-fifths dilated. When they died, he drew on the understanding of the period of the emotional frailty of women as the cause of their deaths.

Johnston never wrote of how the forceps abraded and tore the delicate surface of the vaginal canal, creating the perfect site for life-threatening infection to enter in, nor that the death was an agonising one in which a woman remained conscious and in acute pain almost to the end. His hypothesis and his clinical records of almost 800 women subjected to this practice generated an extended debate in 1873 by the Dublin Obstetrical Society. These scientists meandered around outcomes and numbers. No one, not one scientist, considered the point of how the use of forceps this way might contribute to puerperal fever nearly 40 years after the aetiology of puerperal fever and the need for antisepsis had been established definitively by Semmelweiss and Holmes.

Truth is made operational at many levels by the discourses which have the most power to win legitimacy. There is a keen awareness of contest in this: of battle, of struggle. As Foucault writes, 'Truth is essentially part of a relationship of force' (2003: 53) with the end objective for the winning truth being to present itself as neutral, universal, generalisable. No. 12's truths: of how she became pregnant, where her first child was, how she resolved that she must leave her home (where if she had felt able to give birth, she might well have lived, having no forceps applied to her), her friendless time in Dublin, her lying-in and death, have not counted. Needless to say, there was no inquest.

Maternal death: Twentieth-century institutions, twenty-first-century realities

Throughout the twentieth century, maternal mortality fell dramatically in countries that are termed 'developed economies'. A superstructure of govern-mentality came to bear on maternal health: overarching state policies about the adequacy of maternal health were accompanied by a major expansion of medical research alongside new drugs and technologies. In the UK, the NHS from 1948 onward offered state-funded maternity care free at the point of use. Although this did not pertain in Ireland, where maternity care for all was not free until 1991, the Irish obstetric establishment, like that in the UK and elsewhere, was keen from the mid-twentieth century onward to promote itself as advancing science and technology to make birth 'safer', specifically through the active management of labour associated with the National Maternity Hospital. These proliferating bodies and structures retained all the old problems of hierarchy and power about birth, albeit in new guises.

Embedded in this period of high modernity was a commitment by the state to welfare in the broadest sense, even if differently interpreted by different national governments. This tenet of state responsibility contributed to the establishment in 1952 in the UK of the National Confidential Enquiry Into Maternal Deaths, reporting directly to the Minister for Health. The enquiry became a prized instru-ment viewed the world over as the gold standard of monitoring and surveillance of fatal maternal incidents: careful review by a national body could identify common themes and seek, for example, to lower the numbers of direct maternal deaths due to sepsis. The machinery of the national confidential enquiry led to a kind of security about such scrutiny, trusted by institutions and clinicians in con-sidering how a maternal death had occurred. The emphasis on confidentiality appeared to encourage a practical commitment, so that what had been missed could be identified and responded to without opprobrium. It was of its time: a purely professional undertaking within a hierarchy of governmentality with no direct voice for families. However, to its credit, by the late 1990s the national confidential enquiry had begun to consider in detail the contexts of women's lives: social and economic marginality, domestic violence, mental ill-health after child-birth leading to suicide, the uncertain status of a woman being a migrant or a refugee of minority ethnic status, and how these detrimental factors might impact on a woman's physical and mental well-being as a pregnant and new mother.

Unfortunately, much else was unravelling by then. A diminished sense of public responsibility became apparent as the state contracted out more and more of its core activities to so-called arms-length bodies who tended to squabble among themselves to defend their perceived territory. What we have come to term the hollowing out of the state was well in train. In the UK, the NHS was heading into a permanent crisis of underfunding and great swathes were marketised and handed over to private contractors; an accelerating trend following the 2012 Health and Social Care Act. Successful challenges by birth activists to the direction of mainstream research and policies had gained substantial ground, including the provision of stand-alone midwifery-led units, community-based midwifery, and increased resources for home births. Now these spaces were closing down even as outstanding new research supported their existence.

Maternal death rates among the most marginalised and vulnerable began to rise while the national confidential enquiry itself had become part of the 'enterprise state' subject to competitive tender. In the 2000s, the numbers of maternal deaths in London grew appreciably compared with the rest of the UK (Bewley and Helleur 2012): worsening demographic factors and worsening maternity service provision were intersecting with lethal impact. Northwick Park Hospital in London had ten maternal deaths of minority ethnic women between 2002 and 2005 and was investigated independently and put under special measures (Health-care Commission, 2006). The head of that task force was an obstetrician we would come to know in Ireland in the wake of Savita Halappanavar's death in 2012: Professor Arulkumaran, who was called in by the HSE when the legal team representing her widower objected strenuously to an 'internal' investigation of Savita's death carried out by doctors from Galway University Hospital where she had died.

The myth, recycled by our head of government as late as 2014, was that Ireland had the safest and finest maternity services in the world (The Journal.ie, 2014), a myth actively promulgated by a consultant obstetric establishment that had grown comfortable on double income streams of immensely well-remunerated private practice (with higher rates of unaccountable interventions; see Lutomski et al., 2014) and public salaries. This fiction of best maternity care was maintained by the simple device of not fully counting: the result of flawed mechanisms in ascertaining what constituted a maternal death. Two senior obstetricians deserve praise for becoming increasingly concerned about this haphazard response amid overburdened and seriously underfunded services and who queried this in 2007 (Murphy and O'Herlihy, 2007). Our Department of Health subsequently requested to join the revamped national confidential enquiry in the UK. It was then we discovered that we were average at best (Maternal Death Enquiry, 2012). The statistics themselves became an uncomfortable source of truth.

Creating a dissensus to challenge the state

By 2011, Bimbo had been dead for a year. I had written at once in 2010 to the Master of the hospital where she had come to grief (all three Dublin maternity hospitals retain that title for their clinical head), reminding him of the deaths in London's Northwick Park of vulnerable minority ethnic women, and asking him to bear in mind the concerns of the Nigerian community in Dublin who needed reassurance about a public inquest for Bimbo.[1] With no word twelve months later, of either an inquest or any form of public investigation, I wrote a second letter. Clearly more needed to be done than writing letters. Working with a formidable human rights legal team who gave their time pro bono, and with other help from innumerable sources, it took us two years: to prepare a report based on Bimbo's autopsy record to argue the case for an inquest (on the basis of hospital reports, there had already been a decision that no inquest was required); to locate her widower who had moved to England with their daughter, then aged nine, who had been born with cerebral palsy in another Irish maternity hospital and who herself died ten months after her mother; to raise funds to bring her widower to Dublin; to obtain a visa for him; to find an international obstetric expert on maternal death to advise us; and to ask the independent TD Clare Daly to raise successive questions on the floor of the Dáil to the Minister for Justice about the pressing need for an inquest into Bimbo's death.

Under 1962 legislation, the legal mechanism of a coroner's inquest is not compulsory for maternal deaths and can only be granted by a coroner after due consideration. In reaching a decision, coroners rely on hospital reports. These hospitals have much to lose by way of prestige and reputation. We learned from parliamentary questions lodged by Clare Daly that between 2007 and 2015 the State Claims Agency, acting for hospitals, paid €66 million in legal fees arising from cases involving serious injury and death to either or both women and babies. Payouts for damages totalled €282,883,052, many times more than the total running costs for the maternity services as a whole.

Savita's death was shocking and received such an avalanche of international coverage that an inquest, sought at once by her widower's solicitors, was quickly scheduled for April 2013. It revealed a number of troubling matters to the public. A coroner is an independent legal officer and should also be a medical doctor, and Savita's inquest was a model for how a legal officer's forensic scrutiny can lay bare complex actions, interactions and non-actions in a broken system of care.

We anxiously awaited the conclusion to Bimbo's inquest. On a dark November evening in 2013, after four taxing days of hearings spread over eight months, the Dublin coroner ruled that Bimbo's death was the result of medical misadventure and that her death certificate would be reissued to state this as cause of death. In the gallery, we wept. There was truth at last, not the version of 'truth' which is part of the 'coercive power' that sustains regimes seeking to deny the full experiences of women – as the officials and politicians in the Department of Health and Children, the HSE and the hospitals themselves have consistently done – but the truth of how a beautiful young healthy woman had met her death.

Still our work was not finished. In the autumn of 2012, we faced the reality of six maternal deaths in quick succession, with inquests for only two women. The students argued that the deaths were but the tip of the iceberg, that there were too many near misses; basic care, lacking continuity and affected by cutbacks, on top of all the unresolved historical impasses, was deteriorating. In the autumn of 2014, there were a further three inquests, all with verdicts of medical misadventure. Counting was not enough either.

We started knitting. Students came to lectures with small squares knitted by them, by their grannies, mothers, and children. A project, the Elephant Collective, was taking shape that would draw on people's knitted contributions across the country and beyond. We made contact with the widowers. A committed documentary-maker volunteered to make a film, which included interviews with several widowers (see Chapter 13). The artist who was part of the collective began to paint portraits of the eight women whose families had fought for inquests, all ending in verdicts of medical misadventure (see Chapter 14). Very skilled knitters took the squares and transformed them into a quilt with a design that evoked the absent space of the women who had never returned home, bordered by the protective space they should have had. We were committed to raising public consciousness about maternal deaths and to seeking a new law.

Clare Daly introduced a private member's bill in the Dáil in 2015 to reform the 1962 Coroners Act with an amendment making inquests mandatory for all maternal deaths. The bill had its second reading in December 2015 but progress was maddeningly slow. A chance viewing of our *Picking Up the Threads* exhibition by a Clare county councillor, Mary Howard, led her to put forward and get accepted a motion of support for the legislation by the council, and this opened up yet another space for us. Within six months we had campaigned with most of the remaining county councils and local authorities who followed suit with similar unanimous motions of support forwarded to the government.

On the 23 May 2017, the Minister for Justice, overcoming her former hesitations, announced a separate stand-alone bill to make all maternal deaths subject to mandatory inquests with full compellability of all witnesses and all sources of information, and to make legal aid available to families; the latter a specific need articulated by Clare Daly and her staff who had worked tirelessly within the Dáil for this bill. A tiny fragment of state machinery would be amended thereby annulling the effects of power in other quarters, privileging the voices of families who had hitherto struggled to be heard.

This project has invoked the truth-teller, the *parrhesiastes* who speaks the truth in the most direct and simple way possible to those above, to those in power, to those who would deny truth at all costs to protect themselves (Foucault, 2001). It has effectively challenged several of the rationalities of the Irish state and its institutional and professional networks. Accounts of why women die will now be fully in the public domain.

The project has taught the student midwives from that morning in 2010, all long-qualified, and all the students who have followed after them, how a democratic politics can emerge from their very act of speaking ethically, collectively; of assuming that one has as equal a right to speak as those in the hierarchical order who would otherwise prevent you from speaking. It is this which creates a dissensus (Rancière, 2007), a stance of principled resistance which decentres and challenges that hierarchy, so that it cedes power.

With support across all party lines, our bill will be law by the end of 2017.

Note

1 The Rotunda Hospital in its annual clinical reports recorded thirteen maternal deaths between 2009 and 2013 (Hunter, 2014). Only one went to inquest and there was no other public investigation into these deaths. Important active strategies to reduce maternal deaths have arisen in the UK, outwith the current MBRRACE national confidential enquiry framework. In 2015 the London Maternity Clinical Network set up the London-wide Maternal Mortality Network to collect and share fine-grained data on maternal deaths, while in Scotland the Royal College of Physicians and Surgeons has issued teaching videos to help clinicians to more thoroughly assess unwell women in pregnancy, labour and the postpartum period, with a concentration, above all, on listening to what women are saying.

PART IV
Looking ahead and back

16

CONFRONTING THE STATE OF EMERGENCY WHICH IS OUR MATERNITY SERVICES

Jo Murphy-Lawless, Rosemary Mander and Nadine Edwards

What we call progress is *this* storm.

Walter Benjamin, On the Concept of History

By way of the conclusions we are able to draw from the contributions to this book, certain messages resonate loud, clear and often. Although the authors of the individual chapters have a wide range of personal, occupational and national backgrounds, their messages are shared ones, addressing issues common to all involved with and affected by the damaging conditions which form our contemporary maternity services.

At the heart of this book is our concern, to the point of distress, about the care eked out to childbearing women, their babies and families. The overall well-being of a society can be measured by the quality of the health care it gives. By that measure, the maternity services have been shown to fall seriously short in providing the care to which women are entitled. This shortfall in no way reflects midwives' personal limitations. It is due to the failure or brokenness of defective health care systems and for all the diktats they issue, the failures appear to be no one's responsibility and so the services drift on regardless of the damage. Midwives' experiences, which are recounted here, demonstrate their role to be one of propping up these malfunctioning organisations at immense personal cost. Midwives are clearly made to put at risk not only their own health and social well-being but the gift of their professional skills and their very livelihoods. They have an all-too-clear recognition of the way these systems undermine their ability to provide optimum care and yet they are still prepared, able and motivated to try. This is why we need to take these systems on as our democratic responsibility.

A crucial aspect of the systematic attack (and we cannot call it anything less) on the midwife's role relates to the systematic reduction in the agency of individual midwives by the plethora of institutional, managerial and medical superstructures that control the circumstances of how they must care for childbearing women. Thus, just as the woman's agency has been virtually eliminated by the everyday workings of these structures, the midwife's role has been diminished and downgraded to the point of powerlessness.

The ensuing chaos and turmoil to which this book has drawn attention have for far too long passed unremarked by the agencies who are supposed to have responsibility for the maternity services. The muteness of the institutional, regulatory and governmental superstructure has been deafening. Responses, if any, by these bodies have involved little more than what has become their inevitable knee-jerk reaction, waving about the familiar cover story of 'risk'. Questions about the risk of what and to whom remain unanswered, leading to little more than increasing defensiveness in practice and policymaking, and to palpable fear on the part of women and midwives. Yet all the gaping holes are wrapped up in the continuing deceit highlighting 'progress'.

As contributors to this book, we see it as an urgent requirement to halt this nonspeaking and to break the silence about the real state of affairs.

When the philosopher Walter Benjamin wrote about Paul Klee's picture *Angelus Novus* in 1940, he described a storm so great blowing around this hapless angel of history that a torrent of debris is flung into the very sky: 'What we call progress is *this* storm' (Benjamin, 2003: 392). Benjamin imagines that the angel longs to return to the past in order 'to make whole what was smashed' but the storm of progress is driving him 'irresistibly' into a chaotic future. Several of our contributors have written explicitly of the 'irresistible logic' of our maternity care systems and that irresistibility is implicit in all the other painful contradictions recounted by midwives and women throughout our book. Connecting Benjamin's writing to our case, we can see that these systems drive women and midwives towards a future of birth that fits with our technical, instrumental society: that the future will be but an intensification of the risk protocols and their accompanying algorithms, which already suffocate what should be the living relationship between a woman and her midwife.

The wisdom for us in what Benjamin writes is that we cannot make whole what has already been smashed, but we can see from more than a century of 'organised' professional midwifery (Donnison, 1977) that it has been weighted from the outset to work in tandem with technocratic birth. As matters stand, it is part and parcel of that organisation of modernity which is 'designed to make human actions immune from what the actors believe and feel privately' (Bauman, 1994: 10). This is why we now need to view twentieth-century professional midwifery in all its loss and pain as a history which 'flashes up at a moment of danger' (Benjamin, 2003: 391).

Having reached this moment of danger, how are we to turn towards a more emancipatory project for women and midwives? How do we begin?

Wendy Brown, writing more generally of the crises which confront our contemporary society, tells us that the 'quintessentially *political* question – the question that is both politically relevant and politically responsible – is not "What do you believe in?" but "What is to be done … given who and where we are in history and culture?"' (Brown, 2001: 94).

The actions which must now be taken are political in the sense of thinking differently about individual need and collective response; certainly not to go near the conventional reformist agenda within the existing institutions which have failed so dramatically. Instead we must start from the outside, from the ground up. We must draw on the 'potentialities of ordinary citizens' to discover our 'common concerns' (Wolin, 1994: 11) about birth and the best ways for protecting the midwife–mother relationship. What all the research tells us is that in the right climate women flourish as do the midwives who support them. Our contributors lay bare the towering obstacles to this straightforward relationship. We need to identify each of these obstacles in specific ways to confront and overturn them. For this we will need a vigorous democratic politics that learns from movements like the environmental and ecology campaigns and from social actions in other areas of deep concern, for example responding to the plight of young refugees without basic health care, or building effective low-cost accommodation for homeless families and women experiencing domestic violence. Actions like those taken by the Doctors of the World clinic in London, staffed by volunteer doctors and nurses, show us how to move beyond the official organisations and their usual strictures about what can or should be done or, as they most commonly tell us, cannot be done. Our responses will also need to include the direct actions which come from sophisticated political resistance movements regionally and nationally across the world contesting such core issues as racism and unbridled militarism.

If it is grounded in democratic principles, it can be done. It may also be the most professionally responsible action: using that classic Irish tool of boycott, for example, when understaffing is so great on that day, on that ward, in that unit, that 'care' has become dangerous. A two-hour sit-down boycott in front of the hospital CEO's office (with a press statement sent over social media about the conditions) becomes a vital public duty to protect the well-being of pregnant and labouring women.

Two principles underpin this democratic politics, which are likely to prove uncomfortable at the outset:

- an equality of voice that rejects and rigorously questions the conventional hierarchical order
- an unconditional ethics of 'being there' for the woman.

These appear simple and in many ways they are. They are also immensely threatening and destabilising to existing institutions, which is why we are pressured at all turns to water them down or even drop them altogether. They are fundamental to health services that truly value a country's people, and which are prepared to turn away from the anti-democratic thrust that otherwise seeks to make profit out of the need people have for good care.

So the third requirement we have is to learn how to build a collective dissenting space. Another way to put this is that we need a space 'where the people take up their own equality' (May, 2010: 107) and build a dissensus, which in its demands resists the institutional imperatives to salvage the business-as-usual organisation of the maternity services. We need these spaces to take shape in many different settings on pressing matters about the maternity services, from local communities to the national parliamentary stage.

What might this look like in concrete terms?

Lessons from the Mid Staffs scandal

One example comes from the horrendous Mid Staffordshire Hospital scandal, leading to the deaths from poor care of an estimated 400 to 1,200 patients between 2005 and 2009. It has become a byword for neglect and has raised fundamental questions about how the relations of caring work were brought so low, ending in tragedy for patients and their families. The Mid Staffs scandal is also one of the most thoroughly investigated in recent decades, with five separate reports between 2009 and 2013; two of them conducted by the chair of the final major public inquiry, Sir Robert Francis. In both his first and final reports, for which extensive testimony was taken from all involved, including patients' relatives and staff, Francis cited that among the principal factors contributing to the debacle were poorly resourced structures, sub-standard and non-responsive management, and a chronic shortage of staff (Francis, 2010, 2013). He also stated that in the Mid Staffs climate, bullying had played a major role in enforcing silence on concerned staff who attempted to raise urgent concerns, while family members were disregarded as a matter of course.

It is the families of those who died who took up their own equality and built the collective dissenting space that coalesced in the demand for a full public inquiry and the government's conceding to that demand after earlier inquiries had either been limited officially in their remit, as with the first Francis report, or hedged in by the usual vested interests and regulatory bodies.

A concrete outcome from the second Francis report is a recommendation that has since become law: the statutory duty of candour which requires all health care providers to discuss with people and their families when care goes wrong and harm accrues to the individual. This would not have happened if families had not dug in and resisted, fighting for that public inquiry as Liverpool families fought for the Hillsborough inquest.

A second outcome stems from the many testimonies to the Francis inquiry about the extent of the bullying of individuals who tried to raise concerns, some even being driven into resigning their posts. This resulted in another independent review chaired by Sir Robert Francis called Freedom to Speak Up (Francis, 2015). The accounts that formed part of this last inquiry exposed the depth of the climate of fear within the NHS, the impulse to embed the blame culture still further, and the extremely limited recourse available through existing legislation and regulatory bodies to gain redress and protection for a whistle-blower trying to bring unsafe care out into the open. In his summary, Francis admits that options are limited but hopes that a more open, safety-oriented culture can take root over time, although he does not mention, for instance, the continuing adversities of austerity economics and how these will make it very difficult indeed to have any sustained culture of safety. However, the report is helpful in getting the issue legitimised nationally. At the same time, we need to recognise that systems are self-protective and it is not in their interests to give up bullying tactics and the many ways that poor care can be covered up, so they will try to comply as minimally as possible with any legal constraints, such as they are.

Again it falls to the collective space sustained by a democratic politics to see this matter differently and to hold a different space in order to bring people together to break the toll of suffering on the deliberately targeted, deliberately isolated individual midwife and to expose on her behalf the institutional denials that lie behind tear-stained practice documentation.

This is a space which needs to be both calm and safe. It also needs to be outwith the institutions and their monitoring networks for obvious reasons. A recent and crucial development for midwives and student midwives that fulfils these criteria is online support for those experiencing bullying. There are a number of links including an active Say No to Bullying in Midwifery group and various summary documents, with advice based on experience. Out of this network arose a national Bullying in Midwifery conference held in 2017.

We need many similar networks and endeavours and people also need to become well acquainted with mechanisms such as freedom of information requests, protected disclosures, and parliamentary questions, the last filed through committed parliamentarians who are prepared to work in tandem with local communities. Communities need access to aggregate information from local health authorities on birth outcomes and birth interventions and they need to learn where and who to target to demand better birth facilities and health resources, and how to take court action to pursue those who refuse to respond to evidence and need.

Conclusion

Institutional and political decisions will continue to be made that will have adverse consequences for the care of pregnant women and new mothers and which will adversely affect the working climate and lives of midwives. These institutional decisions are too intimately tied to our crisis-ridden governments that are riven with competing blocs of power and privilege not to succumb to 'crisis-management frenzy' (Bauman, 1993: 211). So conflict is inevitable. Chantal Mouffe (2013) argues that the conflict itself is useful because it is part of an open-ended 'agonistic' democratic politics, with our language to the fore, as distinct from a co-opted consensus politics where we must conform to a vocabulary already set in favour of the very institutions whose practices we are contesting. A language in our terms of reference helps to force change in the direction we need.

Political connectedness will come from these agonistic/democratic politics.

This is ours to take, ours to create.

AFTERWORD

'Mrs Brown is fully'

Rosemary Mander

How do I begin to reflect on almost half a century of being a midwife?

Do I don my rose-tinted spectacles and argue that everything in the garden was lovely when I started and now midwifery is heading for hell in a handcart?

Or do I write about the bad old days of inflexible and unnecessary routines such as the shave, enema and bath for women embarking on normal labour, or the 'OBE' (castor oil, bath and enema) to 'induce' labour?

Perhaps I should aim for a balanced approach, showing a nuanced picture so that we may contemplate and maybe even learn from what has gone before. In this afterword I consider some of the aspects of midwifery and the maternity services that have mattered to me, which have affected what I have done and, hence, may carry implications for others.

The quotation which I have chosen as my title helps us to focus on some of the changes in midwifery. It comprises the words of a much-admired midwife friend and colleague. This was her way of communicating *sotto voce* to midwives practising alongside her in the days of irresistible routines. Her phrase indicated that there was a pot of tea ready, and maybe a few biscuits, cakes or even egg sandwiches. Crucially, though, along with the scrumptious nourishment came the even more valuable sharing of experiences, problems and helpful support. Although such collegial support was widely available, it was only later that the significance of midwives' support for childbearing women became recognised (Mander, 2001).

The routines which I have already mentioned included the iniquitous scheduled induction of labour at 38 weeks' gestation as well as the OBE and its modification for 'preparation' for physiological labour. Such routines have subsequently been recognised as the medicalisation of childbearing and they have become obsolete; their demise was partly due to research findings, such as those of Romney and Gordon (1981). But even more significantly these changes have been associated with a vocal women's lobby, through organisations including what were first known as the Society for the Prevention of Cruelty to Pregnant Women (now AIMS) and the Natural Childbirth Trust (now NCT). Similarly, routine episiotomy has thankfully bitten the dust with the help of more authoritative research by midwives and others (Banta and Thacker, 1982; Sleep *et al.*, 1984). While child-bearing women and midwives would be right to celebrate the demise of such routines, it is necessary to remember that these, at one time standard, iatrogenic interventions have been supplanted by others with a possibly even greater potential for damage (Mander, 2007).

At the same time as women's groups have been crucial in fostering the changes in maternity, midwives have also undergone some quite marked transformations. This may be partly credited to the Association of Radical Midwives (ARM, 2017), whose origins in 1976 followed on from two students' disappointment and frus-tration at what they perceived to be increasing levels of intervention and medicalisation in the care of childbearing women. A mutual support group deve-loped, together with a regular publication, *Midwifery Matters*. The group sought to offer not only support but also change through facilitating the return of midwifery practice to its woman-oriented origins. While not a large group, ARM articulates the values to which many midwives aspire and has been pivotal in encouraging midwives to rethink and reform their roles and loyalties. Such a rethink may be linked with the arrival, development and possible decline of the independent midwife (IM). By providing a novel service of a supremely high, even gold, standard, the IMs have presented other midwives with a benchmark by which to evaluate their practice. Like many of the woman-oriented developments to which I have referred, innovative forms of midwifery practice have not invariably been welcomed by health care providers (Davies and Edwards, 2010).

Some of these changes that I have witnessed may have been facilitated by the developments in midwifery education. Having often been little more than an optional extra after the completion of nurse 'training' (Mander, 1987), midwifery programmes have moved into higher education and now appeal to a more mature and experienced population of, largely, women. Thus, the student as just 'a pair of hands' has become historical. This change in midwifery education is not without its problems and detractions, though. There seem to be phenomenal stress levels for current midwifery students and questions have been raised about the higher education institutions' (HEIs) system of contracting (Humphreys, 1995).

This move into higher education has tended to detach midwife teachers and academics from their clinical colleagues, which may only be prevented by a determined effort of will. But midwife educators and academics have been forced to adopt the values and ethos of the HEIs. These include a focus on research, publications and income-generation, which may all too often be given priority over student contact and support. The significance of research and publication has meant that the growth industry which is midwifery books, journals and on-line materials, has changed out of all recognition from the days when 'Myles', being unique, was regarded as the 'midwife's bible'.

In this way, the blinkered tunnel vision which I encountered when I began in midwifery has, thankfully, moved on. My cross-border activities have made me painfully aware of the huge differences between midwifery practice in Scotland, which at the time was seriously 'over-doctored', and in England, where midwifery practice was more autonomous. Gradually, though, the practice of midwifery in other countries began to have an impact on midwifery in Scotland and England. Initially, in the 1970s the influences were from Ireland through not just the import of Irish students to study midwifery, but through the dogma of the medicalisation of labour through active management (O'Driscoll and Meagher, 1980).

Subsequently, awareness grew of the opportunities open to midwifery through Dutch practice and the exciting developments in New Zealand; but these manifestations of a more autonomous form of midwifery practice proved not to be easily transferable to provide a solution to UK problems. Similarly, we became increasingly aware of the challenges being faced not only in the countries I have mentioned, but also by midwifery and midwives in various forms in North America. In this way midwives' previous narrow outlook was widened, but the extent to which this changing vision has affected practice remains to be seen.

While we are giving credit to remarkable things happening elsewhere, we need to recognise the contribution of the 'giants' whose presence, practice and publications influenced me and which continue to influence midwives. Obviously, my fellow members of the Birth Project Group have been excellent examples. As well as the magnificent role models, we need to recall others whose attitudes and activities were less praiseworthy but who served as the 'grit in the oyster' to encourage a rethink of taken-for-granted assumptions and, thus, changing behaviour.

The changes which I have both witnessed and experienced in the UK National Health Service carry serious implications for the childbearing woman, her family, and, not least, the midwife. In this book we have addressed a wide range of organisational and other developments which cause the midwife to question her ability to provide the care that she knows is needed and only she is able to provide. These changes and developments leave a sense of profound regret that they were not foreseen and, possibly, prevented.

Among these changes are the ensuing changing relationships. The relationship between the woman and baby has been changed by medical technology, meaning that the woman no longer needs to notice the first flutterings in order to report her 'quickening date'. The relationship between the midwife and the woman has similarly changed because there is no longer any reliance on the woman for the last menstrual period date, for reports of fetal movements, and for symptoms of the second stage. Thus, the woman has less authority due to technological investigations, leading to the question of whether the midwife still believes what the woman tells her.

Conclusion

It is clear that childbearing has begun to move away from being a medical event, which it started to become in the 1960s. It is less certain whether this reason for celebration applies to the even more iatrogenically interventive excesses originating in the 1970s.

The nourishing support among midwives has been lost among these and later changes and developments (Pezaro, 2016). It must be a source of concern to anyone who is aware of what is happening in maternity that, rather than being informed that Mrs Brown is fully, the midwife in clinical practice is now more likely to be found ensuring her own physiological functioning by carrying a jug of iced water with a straw.

REFERENCES

Allan J., Fairtlough G. and Heinzen B. (2002) *The Power of the Tale: Using Narratives for Organisational Success*. Chichester: John Wiley.

Allsop J. and Saks M. (2002) *Regulating the Health Professions*. London: Sage.

ARM (2017) Our History. www.midwifery.org.uk/about-us/history (accessed July 2017).

Armstrong F., Clayton L., Crewe J., Edwards N., St Clair A., Seekings-Norman, L. and Wickham S. (2006) The Birth Resource Centre: A Community of Women. In S. Wickham (ed.), *Midwifery Best Practice, Volume 4*. Oxford: Elsevier, 106–11.

Asthana A. (2017) NHS maternity wards in England forced to close 382 times last year. *The Guardian* 8 August 2017. www.theguardian.com/society/2017/aug/08/nhs-maternity-wards-england-forced-closures-labour (accessed 30 Oct 2017).

Aufderheide P. (2007) *Documentary Film: A Very Short Introduction*. New York. Oxford: Oxford University Press.

Auslander P. (1994) Boal, Blau, Brecht: The Body. In M. Schutzman and J. Cohen-Cruz (eds), *Playing Boal: Theatre Therapy Activism*. London: Routledge, 124–33.

Ayers S., Joseph S., McKenzie-McHarg K., Slade P. and Wijma K. (2008) Post-traumatic stress disorder following childbirth: current issues and recommendations for future research. *Journal of Psychosomatic Obstetrics and Gynecology* 29(4): 240–50.

Ayers S., McKenzie-McHarg K., Slade P. (2015) Post-traumatic stress disorder after birth. *Journal of Reproductive & Infant Psychology* 33(3): 215-8.

Baines E. (1983) *The Birth Machine*. London: The Women's Press.

Ball L., Curtis P. and Kirkham M. (2002) *Why do midwives leave?* London: Royal College of Midwives.

Banta D. and Thacker S.B. (1982) The risks and benefits of episiotomy: a review. *Birth* 9(1): 25–30.

Bauman Z. (1993) *Postmodern Ethics*. Oxford: Blackwell.

Bauman Z. (1994) *Alone Again: Ethics after certainty*. London: Demos.

Beattie K. (2004) *Documentary Screens: Nonfiction film and television*. Hampshire: Palgrave Macmillan.

Beck C.T., Logiudice J. and Gable R.K. (2015) A Mixed-Methods Study of Secondary Traumatic Stress in Certified Nurse-Midwives: Shaken Belief in the Birth Process. *Journal of Midwifery & Women's Health* 60(1): 16–23.

Beck U. (1992) *Risk Society: Towards a New Modernity*. London: Sage.

Benjamin W. (2003) *Selected Writings Volume 4, 1938–1940*. Cambridge: Belknap Press of Harvard University Press.

Betterton R. (1996) *Intimate Distance: Women artists and the body*. London: Routledge.

Bewley S. and Helleur A. (2012) Rising maternal deaths in London UK. *The Lancet* 379 (9822): 1198.

Bhatia A. (2015) *Discursive Illusions in Public Discourse*. Abingdon: Routledge.

Bickhoff L., Levett-Jones T. and Sinclair P.M. (2016) Rocking the boat – nursing students' stories of moral courage: A qualitative descriptive study. *Nurse Education Today* 42: 35–40.

Bickhoff L., Sinclair P.M. and Levett-Jones T. (2017) Moral courage in undergraduate nursing students: A literature review. *Collegian* 24: 71–83.

Biello D. (2017) *Inside the debate about power posing: a Q and A with Amy Cuddy*. https://ideas.ted.com/inside-the-debate-about-power-posing-a-q-a-with-amy-cuddy/ (accessed 30 October 2017).

Birthrights (2013) *Dignity in Childbirth: Birthrights Dignity Survey 2013: Women's and midwives' experiences of dignity in UK maternity care*. www.birthrights.org.uk/aboutus/publications (accessed 19 June 2017).

Boal A. (1979) *Theatre of the Oppressed*. London: Pluto.

Boal A. (1992) *Games for Actors and Non-Actors*. London: Routledge.

Boath E., Good R., Tsaroucha A., Stewart T., Pitch S. and Boughey A.J. (2017) Tapping your way to success: using Emotional Freedom Techniques (EFT) to reduce anxiety and improve communication skills in social work students. *Social Work Education*. www.tandfonline.com/doi/full/10.1080/02615479.2017.1297394 (accessed 12 July 2017).

Boyle D. (2011) *The Human Element: Ten new rules to kick-start our failing organisations*. London: Routledge.

BPG (2015) Fear Among Midwives. *RCM* Midwives *Magazine* 82: 60–62.

BPG (2016) Coded rhetoric: The reality of midwifery practice. *British Journal of Midwifery* 24(5): 344–52.

BPG (2017) Birth Project Group. http://pregnancyandparents.org.uk/birth-project-group (accessed July 2017).

Brandimonte M. A., Bruno N. and Collina S. (2006) Cognition. In P. Pawlik and G. d'Ydewalle (eds), *Psychological Concepts: An International Historical Perspective*. Hove: Psychology Press, 11–26.

Brinch S. and Iversen G. (2001) *Reality Images: One hundred years of documentary film*. Oslo: Universitetsforlaget.

Brocklehurst P., Hardy P., Hollowell J., Linsell L., Macfarlane A., McCourt C., Marlow N., Miller A., Newburn M., Petrou S., Puddicombe D., Redshaw M., Rowe R., Sandall J., Silverton L. and Stewart M. (2011) Perinatal and maternal outcomes by planned place of birth for healthy women with low risk pregnancies: the Birthplace in England national prospective cohort study. *BMJ* 343: d7400.

Brodie P. (1996) Australian Team Midwives in Transition. Oslo: International Confederation of Midwives 23rd Triennial Conference.

Broude N. and Garrard M.D. (1996) The Feminist Art Programs at Fresno and CalArts, 1970–75. In N. Broude (eds) *The Power of Feminist Art: The American movement of the 1970s*. New York: Abrams.

Brown W. (2001) *Politics Out of History*. Woodstock: Princeton University Press.

Brydon-Miller M., Kral M., Maguire P., Noffke S. and Sabalok A. (2011) Jazz and the Banyan Tree: Roots and Riffs on Participatory Action Research. In N. K. Denzin and Y. S. (eds), *The Sage Handbook of Qualitative Research, 4th edition*. California: Sage, 387–400.

Bryman A. (2012) *Social Research Methods*. Oxford: Oxford University Press.

Buckley S.J. (2015) Hormonal Physiology of Childbearing: Evidence and Implications for Women, Babies and Maternity Care. Childbirth Connection. A program of the National Partnership for Women & Families. www.nationalpartnership.org/researchlibrary/maternal-health/hormonal-physiology-of-childbearing.pdf (accessed 13 July 2017).

Buurtzorg (2016) www.buurtzorgnederland.com (accessed 12 July 2017).

Campbell D. (2012) NHS watchdog warns of midwife shortage. *The Guardian* 28 June 2012. www.theguardian.com/society/2012/jun/28/midwife-shortage-maternity-units-nhs (accessed 25 July 2017).

Campbell D. (2016) 'Dangerous and unsafe' care driving midwives out of NHS. *The Guardian*, 18 October 2016. www.theguardian.com/society/2016/oct/18/dangerous-and-unsafe-care-driving-midwives-out-of-nhs (accessed 12 July 2017).

Capacitar (2017a) Capacitar training program [Online]. http://capacitar.org/programs (accessed 25 September 2017).

Capacitar (2017b) [Online]. http://capacitar.org/wp-content/uploads/SummerNewsletter 2017_PR.pdf (accessed 25 September 2017).

Capacitar (2017c) Emergency Response Kits [Online]. www.capacitar.org/capacitaremergency-kit (accessed 25 September 2017).

Capacitar (2017d) Manuals and resources [Online]. www.capacitar.org/productcategory/manuals (accessed 25 September 2017).

Carlsson. I.-M., Ziegert K., Sahlberg-Blom E. and Nissen E. (2012) Maintaining power: Women's experiences from labour onset before admittance to maternity ward. *Midwifery* 28(1): 86–93.

Carney D.R., Cuddy A.J.C and Yap A.J. (2010) Power Posing: Brief Nonverbal Displays Affect Neuroendocrine Levels and Risk Tolerance. *Psychological Science* 21(10): 1363–68.

Carolan M. (2011) The good midwife: commencing students' views. *Midwifery* 27(4): 503–8.

Carolan M. (2013) 'A good midwife stands out': 3rd year midwifery students' views. *Midwifery* 29(2): 115–21.

Carolan-Olah M., Kruger G. and Garvey-Graham A. (2015) Midwives' experiences of the factors that facilitate normal birth among low risk women at a public hospital in Australia. *Midwifery* 31(1): 112–21.

Cebulak J.A. (2012) *Midwife Or Med-Wife: Examining Emotion Work with Midwifery Students in Clinical Training.* Master's Thesis, Loyola University Chicago. ProQuest Dissertations Publishing, UMI no 1518459.

Chiarella M. (1995) Regulatory standards: nurses' friend or foe? In G. Gray, R. Pratt (eds) *Issues in Australian Nursing 4.* Pearson Press: Melbourne, 61–74.

Chiarella M. and White J. (2013) Which tail wags which dog? Exploring the interface between professional regulation and professional education. *Nurse Education Today* 33(11): 1274–78.

Chicago J. (1985) *The Birth Project.* New York: Doubleday.

CHRE (2012) *Strategic Review of the Nursing and Midwifery Council: Final Report.* www.professionalstandards.org.uk/docs/default-source/publications/special-review-report/strategic-review-of-nmc-2012.pdf?sfvrsn=2 (accessed June 2015).

Church D., Hawk C., Brooks A.J., Toukolehto O., Wren M., Dinter I. and Stein P. (2013) Psychological trauma symptom improvement in veterans using emotional freedom techniques: a randomized controlled trial. *Journal of Nervous and Mental Disease* 201(2): 153–60.

Cock J. (2014) Sociology and the 'Slow Violence' of Toxic Pollution. *South African Review of Sociology* 45(3): 112–17.

Coldridge L. and Davies S. (2017) 'Am I too emotional for this job?' An exploration of student midwives' experiences of coping with traumatic events in the labour ward. *Midwifery* 45: 1–6.

Collington V., Malik M., Doris F., Fraser D. (2012) Supporting the midwifery practice based curriculum: the role of the link lecturer. *Nurse Education Today* 32(8): 924–9.

Condon J.R. and Cane P.M. (2011) *Capacitar: Healing Trauma, Empowering Wellness.* www.ncdsv.org/images/Capacitar_HealingTraumaEmpoweringWellness_2011.pdf (accessed 12 July 2017).

Cooper J. (2007) *Cognitive Dissonance.* Los Angeles: Sage.

Crowther S., Hunter B., McAra-Couper J., Warren L., Gilkison A., Hunter M., Fielder A. and Kirkham M. (2016) Sustainability and Resilience in Midwifery: A discussion paper. *Midwifery* 40: 40–8.

Cuddy A. (2012) Your body language may shape who you are. [TED talk]. www.ted.com/talks/amy_cuddy_your_body_language_shapes_who_you_are.

Cullen P. (2015) Staff had concerns over problem births at Portiuncula Hospital. *The Irish Times* 24 Jan. www.irishtimes.com/news/health/staff-had-concerns-over-problem-births-at-portiuncula-hospital-1.2077862 (accessed 31 October 2017).

Curtis P., Ball L. and Kirkham M. (2006) Why do midwives leave? (Not) being the kind of midwife you wanted to be. *British Journal of Midwifery* 14(1): 27–31.

Dabrowksi R. (2017) 'Worrying' fall in midwife and nurse numbers. RCM News. www.rcm.org.uk/news-views-and-analysis/news/%E2%80%98worrying%E2%80%99-fall-in-midwife-and-nurse-numbers (accessed 12 July 2017).

Dabrowski R. (2016) New RCM Reports on Staffing. www rcm.org.uk/news-views-andanalysis/news/new-rcm-reports-on-staffing (accessed 20 November 2017).

Dahlen H. (2010) Undone by Fear? Deluded by Trust. *Midwifery* 26(2): 156–62.

Dahlen H.G. and Caplice S. (2014) What do midwives fear? *Women & Birth* 27(4): 266–70.

Dahlen H. and Gutteridge K. (2015) Stop the fear and embrace birth. In S. Byrom and S. Downe (eds) *The Roar Behind the Silence: Why Kindness Compassion and Respect Matter in Maternity Care.* London: Pinter & Martin, 98-104.

Davies L. (2014) The impact of fear of childbirth on the relationship between a mother and her baby. *International Journal of Birth and Parent Education* 1(2): 7–10.

Davies L., Daellenbach R. and Kensington M. (2011) *Sustainability Midwifery and Birth.* London: Routledge.

Davies S. and Coldridge L. (2015) 'No Man's Land': An exploration of the traumatic experiences of student midwives in practice. *Midwifery* 31(9): 858–64.

Davies S. and Edwards N. (2010) Termination of the Albany Practice contract: unanswered questions. *British Journal of Midwifery* 18(4): 260–1.

Deepwell K. (2005) *Dialogues: Women Artists from Ireland.* London: I.B. Tauris.

Deery R. (2010) 'Switching and swapping faces', performativity and emotion in midwifery. *International Journal of Work Organisation and Emotion* 3(3): 272–86.

Deery R. and Kirkham M. (2007) Drained and dumped on: the generation and accumulation of emotional toxic waste in community midwifery. In M. Kirkham (ed) *Exploring The Dirty Side Of Women's Health.* London: Routledge, 72–83.

Devane D., Murphy-Lawless J. and Begley C.M. (2007) Childbirth policies and practices in Ireland and the journey towards midwifery-led care. *Midwifery* 23(1): 92–101.

Diamond D. (1994) Out of Silence: Headlines Theatre and Power Plays. In M. Schutzman and J. Cohen-Cruz (eds) *Playing Boal: Theatre Therapy Activism.* London: Routledge, 35–52.

Dietz S.S. (2016) Using Wordle in qualitative research: a supplemental tool for case studies. *International Journal of Instructional Technology and Distance Learning* 13(8): 23–36.

DoH (1993) *Changing Childbirth: Report of the Expert Maternity Group.* London: HMSO.

DoH (1994) *The Allitt Inquiry: Independent inquiry relating to deaths and injuries on the Children's Ward at Grantham and Kesteven General Hospital during the period February to April 1991: Clothier Report.* London: Department of Health.

DoH (1997) *A First Class Service: Quality in the new NHS.* London: Department of Health.

DoH (2010) *Equity and excellence: Liberating the NHS.* London: Department of Health.

DoH (2012) Health and Social Care Act. Department of Health. London: HMSO. www.legislation.gov.uk/ukpga/2012/7/pdfs/ukpga_20120007_en.pdf (accessed September 2016).

Donnison J. (1977) *Midwives and Medical Men: A History of Inter-Professional Rivalries and Women's Rights.* Ann Arbor, MI: Schocken Press, University of Michigan.

Downe S. (2008) *Normal Childbirth: Evidence and Debate, 2nd edition.* London: Churchill Livingston.

Downe S., McCormick C. and Beech B.L. (2001) Labour interventions associated with normal birth. *British Journal of Midwifery* 9(10): 602–6.

Duffield C., Diers D., O'Brien-Pallas L., Aisbett C., Roche M., King M. and Aisbett K. (2011) Nursing staffing, nursing workload, the work environment and patient outcomes. *Applied Nursing Research* 24(4): 244–55.

Durant E. (2015) *Bullying in midwifery: One small but mighty technique.* Midwife Diaries. www.midwifediaries.com/bullying-in-midwifery (accessed 12 July 2017).

Edwards N. (2014) Pregnancy and Parents Centre. *AIMS Journal* 26(4): 14–5.

Edwards N., Gilbert A., Mander R., McHugh N., Murphy-Lawless J. and Patterson J. (2016) Are staffing shortages changing the culture of midwifery? *The Practising Midwife* 19(3): 12, 14–6.

Edwards N., Murphy-Lawless J., Kirkham M. and Davies S. (2011) Attacks on Midwives, Attacks on Women's Choices. *AIMS Journal* 23(3): 3–6.

Edwards N.P. (2004) Why can't women just say no? And does it really matter? In M. Kirkham (ed.), *Informed Choice in Maternity Care.* Basingstoke: Palgrave Macmillan, 1-29.

Edwards N.P. (2005) *Birthing Autonomy: Women's Experiences of Planning Home Births.* London: Routledge.

Ehrenreich B. and Hochschild A.R. (2002) *Global Woman: Nannies, Maids and Sex Workers in the New Economy.* London: Granta.

Eighth Amendment of the Constitution Act (1983). www.irishstatutebook.ie/eli/1983/ca/8/section/1/enacted/en/html#sec1.

Fahy K.A. (2002) Reflecting on Practice to Theorise Empowerment for Women: Using Foucault Concepts. *The Australian Journal of Midwifery* 15(1): 5–13.

Fairtlough G. (1994) *Creative Compartments: A Design for Future Organisation.* London: Adamantine Press.

Fairtlough G. (2005) *The Three Ways of Getting Things Done: Hierarchy, Heterarchy and Responsible Autonomy in Organisations.* Bridport: Triarchy Press.

Fissell M. (2004) *Vernacular Bodies: The Politics of Reproduction in Early Modern England.* Oxford: Oxford University Press.

Fleming V. (2002) Statutory Control. In R. Mander and V. Fleming (eds), *Failure to Progress: The Contraction of the Midwifery Profession.* London: Routledge, 63-77.

Foucault M. (2001) *Fearless Speech.* Los Angeles: Semiotexte.

Foucault M. (2002) *Power: Essential Works of Foucault 1954–1984, Volume 3.* London: Penguin.

Foucault M. (2003) *Society Must Be Defended: Lectures at the Collège de France 1975–76.* London: Penguin.

Foucault M. (2009) *Security, Territory, Population: Lectures at the Collège de France 1977–78*, M. Sennelart (ed.). Basingstoke: Palgrave Macmillan.

Francis R. (2010) *Independent Inquiry into care provided by Mid Staffordshire NHS Foundation Trust January 2005–March 2009*,Volume I. HC375-I Session 2009/10. London: HMSO.

Francis R. (2013) *Report of the Mid Staffordshire NHS Foundation Trust Public Inquiry*. London: HMSO. www.midstaffspublicinquiry.com/report (accessed August 2016).

Francis R. (2015) *Freedom to Speak Up: An independent review into creating an open and honest reporting culture in the NHS*. www.freedomtospeakup.org.uk/the-report.

Fraser N. (2016) Contradictions of Capital and Care. *New Left Review* 100: 99–117.

Friedenwald-Fishman E. (2011) No Art? No Social Change No Innovation Economy. Stanford Social Innovation Review. https://ssir.org/articles/entry/no_art_no_social_change._no_innovation_economy (accessed 3 January 2017).

Gaines J. (1999) *Collecting Visible Evidence*. Minneapolis: University of Minnesota Press.

Garlick H. (2016) Labour of love: the volunteers helping fellow refugees give birth. *The Guardian* 17 December. www.theguardian.com/world/2016/dec/17/labour-love-volunteer-doulas-helping-fellow-refugees (accessed 20 July 2017).

Garthus-Niegel S., Soest T., Vollrath M.E. and Eberhard-Gran M. (2013) The impact of subjective birth experiences on post-traumatic stress symptoms: a longitudinal study. *Archives of Women's Mental Health* 16(1): 1–10.

Gaskin I. M. (2008) Maternal Death in the United States: A Problem Solved or a Problem Ignored? *Journal of Perinatal Education* 17(2): 9–13. doi:10.1624/105812408X298336

Geiger J. (2011) *American Documentary Film: Projecting the Nation Edinburgh*. Edinburgh: Edinburgh University Press.

Gillen P., Sinclair M. and Kernohan G. (2008) The nature and manifestations of bullying in midwifery. www.thewisehippo.com/wp-content/uploads/2016/04/University_of-Ulster_The_nature_and_manifestations_of_bullying_in_midwifery_Research_Summary.pdf (accessed 12 July 2017).

Graeber D. (2015) *The Utopia of Rules: On technology, stupidity, and the secret joys of bureaucracy*. London: Melville House.

Greenfield M. (2016) What is traumatic birth? A concept analysis and literature review. *British Journal of Midwifery* 24(4): 254–67.

Greenhalgh T. and Taylor R. (1997) Papers that go beyond numbers. *BMJ* 315: 740-3.

Grehan M. (2007) The Delivery of Art in a Maternity Hospital. In L. Davies (ed.), *The Art and Soul of Midwifery: Creativity in Practice Education and Research*. Edinburgh: Churchill Livingstone, 46–61.

Griffiths J. (2016) Stress affects almost 50% of England's midwives. RCM. www.rcm.org.uk/news-views-and-analysis/news/stress-affects-almost-50-of-englands-midwives (accessed 22 June 2017).

Guarneri E. and King R.P. (2015) Challenges and Opportunities Faced by Biofield Practitioners in Global Health and Medicine: A White Paper. *Global Advances in Health Medicine*, 4 (Suppl.), 89–96. [Online]. www.ncbi.nlm.nih.gov/pmc/articles/PMC4654785.

Guilliland K. and Pairman S. (2011) *Women's Business. The story of the New Zealand College of Midwives 1986–2010*. Christchurch NZ: NZCOM.

Gutierrez K.M. (2005) Critical care nurses' perceptions of and responses to moral distress. *Dimensions of Critical Care Nursing* 24(5): 229–41.

Harding L. (2003) Leni Riefenstahl Hitler's favourite film propagandist dies at 101. *The Guardian* 10 September. www.theguardian.com/world/2003/sep/10/film.germany (accessed 8 December 2016).

Harris K. (2016) Daughters of the Revolution [Audio Podcast], K. Harris producer. http://4elements.ie/post-show-discussion-videos (accessed July 2017).

Harris R. and Ayers S. (2012) What makes labour and birth traumatic? A survey of intrapartum 'hotspots'. *Psychology & Health* 27(10): 1166–77.

Healthcare Commission (2006) *Investigation into 10 maternal deaths at or following delivery at Northwick Park Hospital North West London Hospitals NHS Trust between April 2002 and April 2005.* London: Commission for Healthcare Audit and Inspection.

Heritage P. (2004) Taking Hostages: Staging human rights. *The Drama Review* 48 (3): 96–106. doi: 10.1162/1054204041667695.

Hinegardner L. (2009) Action, Organization and Documentary Film – Beyond a Communications Model of Human Rights Videos. *Visual Anthropology Review* 25(2): 172–85.

HMSO (1858) *An Act to Regulate the Qualifications of Practitioners in Medicine and Surgery Chapter 90.* www.legislation.gov.uk/ukpga/Vict/21-22/90/enacted (accessed July 2016).

Hofrichter R. (2000) *Reclaiming the Environmental Debate: The Politics of Health in a Toxic Culture.* Cambridge: MIT Press.

Homer C.S.E., Leap N., Edwards N. and Sandall S. (2017) Midwifery continuity of carer in an area of high socio-economic disadvantage in London: a retrospective analysis of Albany Midwifery Practice outcomes using routine data 1997–2009. *Midwifery* 48: 1–10.

House of Commons Health Committee *(1992) Maternity services Vol I report HC 29-I.* London: HMSO.

Hughes D. (2015) 'Take Two Paracetamol' and Labour. *Midwifery Matters* 145: 14–5.

Hughes D. (2017) Midwives – still eating their young. *Midwifery Matters* 153: 13.

Humphreys J. (1995) Paradigms of Practice: a dilemma for nurse educators. *The Vocational Aspect of Education* 47(2): 113–27.

Hunt S. and Symonds A. (1995) *The Social Meaning of Midwifery.* London: Macmillan Press Ltd.

Hunter B. (2004) Conflicting ideologies as a source of emotion work in midwifery. *Midwifery* 20(3): 261–72.

Hunter B. (2014) One-to-one: Bouncing back. *RCM Midwives Magazine* 2. www.rcm.org. uk/news-views-and-analysis/analysis/one-to-one-bouncing-back (accessed 12 July 2017).

Hunter B., Berg M., Lundgren I., Olafsdottir O. and Kirkham M. (2008) Relationships: The hidden threads in the tapestry of maternity care. Guest commentary. *Midwifery* 24(2): 132–7.

Hunter B. and Warren L. (2013) *Investigating Resilience in Midwifery: Final report.* Cardiff University: Cardiff.

Hunter B. and Warren L. (2014) Midwives' experiences of workplace resilience. *Midwifery* 30(8): 926–34

Hunter N. (2014) 3 maternal deaths at the Rotunda last year. *Irish Healthcom* 2 December 2014. www.irishhealth.com/articlehtml?id=24233.

Hurwitz B. (2008) *The intimate massacre: the Harold Shipman case.* Research seminar paper 2008/09, Cardiff Crime Narratives Network, Cardiff University.

Inglis T. (2003) *Truth, Power and Lies: Irish Society and the Case of the Kerry Babies.* Dublin: UCD Press.

ICM (2017) *Definition of a midwife.* http://internationalmidwives.org/who-we-are/policy-and-practice/icm-international-definition-of-the-midwife

Ireland Department of Health and Children (2016) National Maternity Strategy – Creating a Better Future Together 2016–2026. Dublin. www.health.gov.ie/blog/publications/national-maternity-strategy-creating-a-better-future-together-2016-2026 (accessed July 2017).

Irish Nurses and Midwives Organisation (2014) INMO Midwifery Staffing Survey Confirms Major Staffing Crisis. Press release, 6 March 2014. www.inmo.ie/Home/Index/7896/11582.

Irvine J. (1992) Review: Sounding the Depths. Irish Museum of Modern Art Dublin 1 April–9 April 1992. *CIRCA Arts Magazine* 62: 64–6.

Jackson D., Firtko A. and Edenborough M. (2007) Personal resilience as a strategy for surviving and thriving in the face of workplace adversity: A literature review. *Journal of Advanced Nursing* 60(1): 1–9.

Jacobs J. (1992) *Systems of Survival: A dialogue on the moral foundations of commerce and politics.* London: Hodder and Stoughton.

Jameton A. (1984) *Nursing Practice: The Ethical Issues.* Englewood Cliffs NJ: Prentice-Hall.

Johnston G. (1869) *Clinical Report of the Rotunda Lying-in Hospital for the Year Ending 5th November 1869.* Dublin Quarterly Journal of Medical Science Volume XLIV, February and May 1870, 101–12.

Jones T.L., Hamilton P. and Murry N. (2015) Unfinished nursing care, missed care, and implicitly rationed care: State of the science review. *International Journal of Nursing Studies* 52(6): 1122–37.

Jordanova L. (1989) *Sexual Visions: Images of gender in science and medicine between the eighteenth and twentieth centuries.* Brighton: Harvester Wheatsheaf.

Kahana J. (2008) *Intelligence Work: The Politics of American Documentary.* New York: Columbia University Press.

Kahn J. (1853) *Catalogue of Dr Kahn's Celebrated Anatomical Museum from 315 Oxford Street London. Now exhibiting at the Rotunda Hospital Dublin* (non-listed).

Kelly M. (1983) *Post-Partum Document.* University of California Press: Berkeley.

Kemp M. (1992) True to Their Natures: Sir Joshua Reynolds and Dr William Hunter at the Royal Academy of Arts. *Notes and Records of the Royal Society of London* 46(1): 77–88.

Kienle G.S. and Kiene H. (2011) Clinical judgement and the medical profession. *Journal of Evaluation in Clinical Practice* 17(4): 621–7.

Kirkham M. (1999) The culture of midwifery in the National Health Service in England. *Journal of Advanced Nursing* 30(3): 732–9.

Kirkham M. (2007) Traumatised Midwives. *AIMS Quarterly Journal* 19(1): 12-13. www.aims.org.uk/Journal/Vol19No1/traumatisedMidwives.htm (accessed 20 November 2017).

Kirkham M. (2010) *The Midwife-Mother Relationship 2nd Edition.* Basingstoke Hampshire: Palgrave Macmillan.

Kirkham M. (2017a) A fundamental contradiction: the business model does not fit midwifery values. *Midwifery Matters* 152: 13–5.

Kirkham M. (2017b) Resilience: a lost concept of limited use for midwives. *Midwifery Matters* 152: 6–8.

Kirkham M. (2017c) Fundamental contradiction. *AIMS Journal* 29(1): 6–8.

Kirkham M., Morgan R.K. and Davies C. (2006) *Why Midwives Stay.* London: Department of Health.

Kirkham M., Stapleton H., Thomas G. and Curtis P. (2002) Checking not listening: how midwives cope. *British Journal of Midwifery* 10(7): 447–50.

Kirkup B (2015) *The report of the Morecambe Bay Investigation* UK Government Publications: The Stationery Office, London

Kitzinger J., Green J. and Coupland V. (1990) Labour relations: midwives and doctors on the labour ward. In J. Garcia R. Kilpatrick and R. Richards (eds), *The Politics of Maternity Care.* Oxford: Clarendon Press, 149–62.

Kitzinger S. (2006) *Birth Crisis.* London: Routledge.

Korsmeyer C. (2004) *Gender and Aesthetics: An Introduction.* New York: Routledge.

KPMG (2008) *Independent Review of the Maternity and Gynaecology Services in the Greater Dublin Area.* Dublin: KPMG. www.hse.ie/eng/services/publications/hospitals/

Independent_Review_of_Maternity_and_Gynaecology_Services_in_the_greater_Dubli n_area_.html (accessed 20 November 2017).

Lash S. and Wynne B. (1992) *Introduction. In* U. Beck *Risk Society: Towards a New Modernity*. London: Sage.

Lazzarato M. (2009) Neoliberalism in Action: Inequality, Insecurity and the Reconstitution of the Social Theory. *Culture and Society* 26(6): 109–33.

Leap N. (1997) Making sense of 'horizontal violence' in midwifery. *British Journal of Midwifery* 5(11): 689.

Leap N. (2010) *The Less We Do the More We Give*. In M. Kirkham (ed.), The Midwife-Mother Relationship 2nd Edition. Basingstoke Hampshire: Palgrave Macmillan, 17–36.

Leap N., Sandall J., Buckland S. and Uber U. (2010) Journey to Confidence: Women's Experiences of Pain in Labour and Relational Continuity of Care. *Journal of Midwifery and Women's Health* 55(3): 234–42.

Leinweber J., Creedy D.K., Rowe H. and Gamble J. (2017a) A socioecological model of posttraumatic stress among Australian midwives. *Midwifery* 45: 7–13.

Leinweber J., Creedy D.K. and Rowe H. and Gamble J. (2017b) Responses to birth trauma and prevalence of posttraumatic stress among Australian midwives. *Women and Birth* 30(1): 40–45

Leversidge A. (2016) On employment: Why midwives leave – revisited. RCM News. www.rcm.org.uk/news-views-and-analysis/news/on-employment-why-midwives-leave-%E2%80%93-revisited (accessed 20 November 2017).

Long S. (2008) *The Perverse Organisation and its Deadly Sins*. London: Karnac.

Lundgren I., Karlsdottir S.I. and Bondas T. (2009) Long-term memories and experiences of childbirth in a Nordic context—a secondary analysis. *International Journal of Qualitative Studies on Health and Well-being* 4: 115–28.

Lutomski J.E., Murphy M., Devane D., Meaney S. and Greene R.A. (2014) Private health care coverage and increased risk of obstetric intervention. *BMC Pregnancy and Childbirth* 2014 14:13. doi.org/10.1186/1471-2393-14-13.

Machin D. and Scamell M. (1997) The experience of labour using ethnography to explore the irresistible nature of the bio-medical metaphor during labour. *Midwifery* 13(2): 78–84.

Macintosh K. (2011) Interview: Dr John Gillies. *Holyrood Magazine* 28 January 2011. www.holyrood.com/2011/01/leading-from-the-front (accessed 20 November 2017).

Mackintosh N., Watson K., Rance S. and Sandall J. (2016) I'm left in fear. An Account of Patient Harm in maternity care. In J.K. Johnson, H.W. Haskell and P.R. Barach, *Case Studies in Patient Safety: Foundations for Core Competencies*. Burlington MA: Jones & Bartlett Learning, 63–72.

Maguire M.J. (2001) The Changing Face of Catholic Ireland: Conservatism and Liberalism in the Ann Lovett and Kerry Babies Scandals. *Feminist Studies* 27(2) 335–58.

Mander R. (1987) *The Employment Decisions of Newly Qualified Midwives*. Unpublished PhD thesis, University of Edinburgh.

Mander R. (2001) *Supportive Care and Midwifery*. Oxford: Blackwell Science.

Mander R. (2007) *Caesarean: Just Another Way of Birth?* London: Routledge.

Mander R. (2014) Smoke and mirrors. *Midwives* 17(5): 26.

Mander R. (2016) Coded rhetoric: The reality of midwifery practice. *British Journal of Midwifery* 24(5): 344–52.

Mander R. and Murphy-Lawless J. (2013) *The Politics of Maternity*. London and New York: Routledge.

Mander R. and Fleming V. (2002) *Failure to Progress: The Contraction of the Midwifery Profession*. London: Routledge.

Marmot M. (2016) *The Health Gap: The Challenge of an Unequal World*. London: Bloomsbury.

Massey L. (2005) Pregnancy and Pathology: Picturing Childbirth in Eighteenth-Century Obstetric Atlases. *The Art Bulletin* 87(1): 73–91.

Maternal Death Enquiry (2012) *Confidential Maternal Death Enquiry Report for Triennium 2009–2011*. Cork: MDE.

May T. (2010) *Contemporary Political Movements and the Thought of Jacques Rancière: Equality in Action*. Edinburgh: Edinburgh University Press.

McCafferty N. (1985) *A Woman to Blame: The Kerry Babies Case*. Dublin: Attic Press.

McCourt C. and Stevens T. (2009) Relationship and Reciprocity in Caseload Midwifery. In B. Hunter and R. Deery (eds), *Emotions in Midwifery and Reproduction*. Basingstoke: Palgrave Macmillan, 17–35.

McKenzie-McHarg K., Ayers S., Ford E., Horsch A., Jomeen A., Sawyer A., Stramrood C., Thomson G. and Slade P. (2015) *Post-traumatic stress disorder following childbirth: an update of current issues and recommendations for future research*. *Journal of Reproductive and Infant Psychology* 33(3. doi: 10.1080/02646838.2015.1031646

McLeod S. (2014) Cognitive Dissonance. [Online] www.simplypsychology.org/cognitive-dissonance.html (accessed 20 November 2017).

Morgan K.P (1998) Contested Bodies Contested Knowledges: Women, Health and the Politics of Medicalization. In S. Sherwin (ed.), *The Politics of Women's Health: Exploring Agency and Autonomy*. Philadelphia: Temple University Press, 83-121.

Morris S. (2005) Is fear at the heart of hard labour? *MIDIRS Midwifery Digest* 15(4): 508–11.

Mouffe C. (2013) *Agonistics: Thinking the World Politically*. London: Verso.

Murphy C. and O'Herlihy C. (2007) Maternal Mortality Statistics in Ireland: Should they carry a health warning? *Irish Medical Journal* 100(8): 574.

Murphy-Lawless J. (1988) The Silencing of Women in Childbirth or Let's Hear It from Bartholomew and the Boys. *Women's Studies International Forum* 11(4): 293–8.

Murphy-Lawless J. (1998) *Reading Birth and Death: A History of Obstetric Thinking*. Cork: University Press Cork.

Murphy-Lawless J. (2014) Anything but Simple: Why we need to understand the 2012 Health and Social Care Act. *AIMS Journal* 26(3): 6–11.

Murphy-Lawless J., Mander R., McHugh N. and Edwards N. *Supporting early years meaningfully*. Forthcoming.

Nelson K., Sartwell T. and Rouse D. (2016) Electronic fetal monitoring cerebral palsy and caesarean section: assumptions versus evidence. *BMJ* 355:i6405 doi: 101136/bmji6405.

NHS Choices (2011) Wellbeing self-assessment. www.nhs.uk/Tools/Documents/Wellbeing%20self-assessment.htm (accessed 12 July 2017).

NHS England (2016) National Maternity Review: Better Births. Improving outcomes in maternity services in England. A Five Year Forward View for Maternity Care. Chair Julia Cumberledge. www.england.nhs.uk/mat-transformation/mat-review (accessed 20 November 2017).

NICE (2014) NICE clinical guideline 190 – Intrapartum care: care of healthy women and their babies during childbirth. National Institute for Clinical Effectiveness NICE. www.nice.org.uk/guidance/cg190 (accessed 20 November 2017).

Nicoll A., Hoggins K. and Winters P. (2005) Waterbirth – changing attitudes. *AIMS Journal* 17(4): 12–14.

Nieuwenhuijze M.J., de Jonge A., Korstjens I., Budé L an.d Largo Janssen T.L.M. (2013) Influence on birthing positions affects women's sense of control in second stage of labour. *Midwifery* 29 e107–e114.

Nixon R. (2011) *Slow Violence and the Environmentalism of the Poor*. Cambridge: Harvard University Press.

NMC (2009) *Standards for pre-registration midwifery education.* www.nmc.org.uk/standards/additional-standards/standards-for-pre-registration-midwifery-education (accessed 31 May 2017).

NMC (2015) *The Code: Professional standards of practice and behaviour for nurses and midwives.* Nursing & Midwifery Council London. www.nmc.org.uk/globalassets/sitedocuments/nmc-publications/nmc-code.pdf (accessed August 2016).

NMC (2016a) NMC appoints Professor Mary Renfrew FRSE to lead development of new midwifery standards. Press release, 30 November 2016. www.nmc.org.uk/news/press-releases/nmc-appoints-professor-mary-renfrew-frse-to-lead-development-of-new-mid wifery-standards (accessed 20 November 2017).

NMC (2016b) *Changes to midwifery regulation.* www.nmc.org.uk/about-us/policy/projects-were-involved-in/changes-to-midwifery-regulation (accessed August 2016).

NMC (2017) Indemnity provision for IMUK midwives is 'inappropriate', says NMC. Statement on indemnity scheme provided for IMUK members. Press release 13 January, 2017. www.nmc.org.uk/news/news-and-updates/indemnity-provision-for-imuk-midwives-is-inappropriate-says-nmc/ (accessed 20 November 2017).

Nursing and Midwifery Board of Ireland (2016) New education Standards and Requirements to support nursing and midwifery care. Press release 9 February 2016. www.nmbi.ie/News-Events/News/New-education-Standards-and-Requirements-to-suppor (accessed 20 November 2017).

O'Driscoll K. and Meagher D. (1980) *Active Management of Labour.* London: Saunders.

O'Malley M-P. (2010) 'So either you have a foetal monitor or you have your waters broken, basically is it?' Articulating maternity care policy at a midwives' ante-natal clinic. *Language Policy* 9: 87–96 doi: 10.1007/s10993-009-9152-9.

O'Malley-Keighran M-P. and Lohan G. (2016) Encourages and guides, or diagnoses and monitors: Woman centred-ness in the discourse of professional midwifery bodies. *Midwifery* 43: 48–58.

O'Toole F. (2010) *Enough is Enough: How to Build a New Republic.* London: Faber.

Ormston, R., McConville, S., Gordon, J. (2014) *Evaluation of the Family Nurse Partnership Programme in NHS Lothian Scotland: Summary of Key Learning and Implications.* Edinburgh: Scottish Government Social Research. www.scotland.gov.uk/Resource/0044/0 0444851.pdf (accessed 20 November 2017).

Page M. and Mander R. (2014) Intrapartum uncertainty: A feature of normal birth, as experienced by midwives in Scotland. *Midwifery* 30(1): 28–35.

Pezaro S. (2016) The case for developing an online intervention to support midwives in work-related psychological distress. *British Journal of Midwifery* 24 (11): 799-805.

Pezaro S., Clyne W., Turner A., Fulton E.A. and Gerada C. (2015) 'Midwives Overboard!' Inside their hearts are breaking, their makeup may be flaking but their smile still stays on. *Women and Birth* 29(3): e59–e66.

Pilger J. (2004) *Tell Me No Lies: Investigative Journalism and its Triumphs.* London:Vintage.

Pollock A.M. (2005) *NHS plc 2nd edition.* London and New York:Verso.

Pollock A. and Price D. (2011) How the secretary of state for health proposes to abolish the NHS in England. *BMJ* 342: d1695.

Pollock G. (2009) Mother Trouble: The Maternal-Feminine in Phallic and Feminist Theory in Relation to Bracha Ettinger's Elaboration of Matrixial Ethics/Aesthetics. *Studies in the Maternal* 1(1): 1–32. www.mamsie.bbk.ac.uk (accessed 20 November 2017).

Pollock J. (2015) Unexpected consequences of midwifery in the NHS. *The Practising Midwife* 18(10): 34–6, 38.

Priddis H.S., Keedle H. and Dahlen H. (2017) The Perfect Storm of Trauma: The experiences of women who have experienced birth trauma and subsequently accessed residential parenting services in Australia. *Women and Birth*. www.doi.org/10.1016/j.wombi.2017.06.007.

Prusova K., Churcher L., Tyler A. and Lokugamage, A.U. (2014) Royal College of Obstetricians and Gynaecologists guidelines: how evidence-based are they? *Journal of Obstetrics and Gynaecology* 348: 706–11.

PSA (2016) Professional Standards Authority for Health and Social Care. www.professionalstandards.org.uk (accessed August 2016).

Putz R., O'Hara K., Taggart F. and Stewart-Brown S. (2012) *Using WEMWBS to measure the impact of your work on mental well-being: A practice-based user guide.* www2.warwick. ac.uk/fac/med/research/platform/wemwbs/researchers/userguide (accessed 12 July 2017).

Quashie M. (2015) Fight for rights: a mother's perspective. *The Practising Midwife* 18(9): 50.

Rafferty A.M., Clarke S.P., Coles J., Ball J., James P., McKee M. and Aiken L.H. (2007) Outcomes of variation in hospital nurse staffing in English hospitals: Cross-sectional analysis of survey data and discharge records. *International Journal of Nursing Studies* 44 (2): 175–82.

Rance S., McCourt C., Rayment J., Mackintosh N., Carter W., Watson K. and Sandall J. (2013) Women's safety alerts in maternity care: is speaking up enough? *BMJ Quality and Safety* 224: 348–55.

Rancière J. (2007) *On the Shores of Politics*. London: Verso.

RCM (2016a) *The RCM Standards for Midwifery Services in the UK*. London RCM. www.rcm.org.uk/sites/default/files/RCM%20Standards%20for%20Midwifery%20Services%20in%20the%20UK%20A4%2016pp%202016_12.pdf (accessed 31 May 2017).

RCM (2016b) *Why Midwives Leave – Revisited*. London: RCM. www.rcm.org.uk/sites/default/files/Why%20Midwives%20Leave%20Revisted%20-%20October%202016.pdf (accessed 12 July 2017).

RCM (2016c) *Royal College of Midwives: Caring for You Campaign*. www.rcm.org.uk/caring-for-you-campaign (accessed 13 July 2017).

RCN (2013) *Beyond Breaking Point?* Royal College of Nursing. London. www.rcn.org.uk/professional-development/publications/pub-004448 (accessed April 2015).

RCN (2016) *The Buurtzorg Nederland home care provider model – Observations for the UK*. www.rcn.org.uk/about-us/policy-briefings/br-0215 (accessed 12 July 2017).

Reed B. (2016) *Birth in Focus*. London: Pinter & Martin.

Reed R., Sharman R. and Inglis C. (2017) Women's descriptions of childbirth trauma relating to care provider actions and interactions. *BMC Pregnancy and Childbirth* 17: 21 doi: 101186/s12884-016-1197-0.

Reiger K. and Lane K. (2013) 'How can we go on caring when nobody here cares about us?' Australian public maternity units as contested care sites. *Women and Birth* 26(2): 133–7.

Renfrew M.J., McFadden A., Bastos M.H., Campbell J., Channon A.A., Cheung N.F., Silva D.R.A.D., Downe S., Powell Kennedy H., Malata A, McCormick F., Wick L. and Declercq E. (2014) Midwifery and quality care: findings from a new evidence informed framework for maternal and newborn care. *The Lancet:* 384 (9948): 1129-45. doi: 10.1016/S0140-6736 (14) 60789.

Reynolds E.K., Cluett E. and Le-May A. (2014) Fairy tale midwifery - fact or fiction: The lived experiences of newly qualified midwives. *British Journal of Midwifery* 22(9): 660–8.

Rice H. and Warland J. (2013) Bearing witness: midwives experiences of witnessing traumatic birth. *Midwifery* 29(9): 1056–1063.

Rich A. (1976) *Of Woman Born: Motherhood as Experience and Institution*. New York: W.W. Norton & Co.

Rizq R. (2012) The perversion of care: Psychological therapies in a time of IAPT. *Psychodynamic Practice* 18(1): 7–24.

Roberts S. (2015) Jacob Riis Photographs Still Revealing New York's Other Half. New York Times 22 October. www.nytimes.com/2015/10/23/arts/design/jacob-riis-photographs-still-revealing-new-yorks-other-half.html (accessed 5 December 2016).

Romney M. and Gordon H. (1981) Is your enema really necessary? *BMJ* 282(6272): 1269–71.doi:10.1136/bmj.282.6272.1269.

Rubik B. (2008) Measurement of the Human Biofield and Other Energetic Instruments. www.faim.org/measurement-of-the-human-biofield-and-other-energetic-instruments (accessed 12 July 2017).

Sackler E.A. (2002) *Judy Chicago*. New York: Watson-Guptil Publications.

Saks M. (2014) Regulating the English healthcare professions: Zoos, circuses or safari parks? *Journal of Professions and Organization* 1(1): 84–98.

Salverson J. (1994) The Mask of Solidarity. In M. Schutzman, J. Cohen-Cruz (eds), *Playing Boal: Theatre Therapy Activism*. London: Routledge, 157–70.

Sandall J. (1998) Occupational burnout in midwives: new ways of working and the relationship between occupational factors and psychological health and wellbeing. *Risk Decision and Policy* 3(3): 213–32.

Sandall J., Coxon K., Mackintosh N., Rayment-Jones H., Locock L. and Page L. writing on behalf of the Sheila Kitzinger symposium. (2016) *Relationships: the pathway to safe high-quality maternity care. Report from the Sheila Kitzinger Symposium*, Oxford. www.gtc. ox.ac.uk/images/stories/academic/skp_report.pdf (accessed 26 May 2017).

Sandall J., Soltani H., Gates S., Shennan A. and Devane D. (2016) *Midwife-led continuity models versus other models of care for childbearing*. Cochrane Database of Systematic Reviews Issue 4 Art. No. CD004667.

Scamell M. and Stewart M. (2014) Time, risk and midwife practice: the vaginal examination. *Health, Risk and Society* 16(1): 84–100.

Scherkenbach W.W. (1986) *Quality and Productivity: Road Maps and Road Blocks*. London: Mercury.

Schiebinger L. (1993) *Nature's Body: Gender in the Making of Modern Science*. Boston: Beacon Press.

Schroeder E., Stavros P., Patel N., Hollowell J., Puddicombe D., Redshaw M. and Brocklehurst P. (2012) Cost effectiveness of alternative planned places of birth in women at low risk of complications: evidence from the Birthplace in England national prospective cohort study. *BMJ* 344: e2292.

Schroeder L., Patel N., Keeler M. and Macfarlane A. (2017) The economic costs of intrapartum care in Tower Hamlets: a comparison between the cost of birth in a freestanding midwifery unit and hospital for women at low risk of obstetric complications. *Midwifery* 45: 28-35.

Schutzman M. (1994) Brechtian Shamanism. In M. Schutzman, J. Cohen-Cruz (eds). *Playing Boal: Theatre Therapy Activism*. London: Routledge, 137–56.

Scottish Government (2017) The Best Start: A Five-Year Forward Plan for Maternity and Neonatal Care in Scotland. www.gov.scot/Resource/0051/00513175.pdf.

Secretary of State for Health (2003) The Shipman Inquiry, Third Report, CM5854. London: Crown Copyright. www.gov.uk/government/uploads/system/uploads/attachment_data/file/273227/5854.pdf (accessed August 2016).

Shallow H. (2001) Competence and confidence: Working in a climate of fear. *British Journal of Midwifery* 9(4): 237–44.

Shallow H.E.D. (2016) *Are you listening to me? An exploration of the interactions between mothers and midwives when labour begins. A Feminist Participatory Action Research Study*. Unpublished PhD, University of the West of Scotland.

Sheen K., Spiby H. and Slade P. (2015) Exposure to traumatic perinatal experiences and post-traumatic stress symptoms in midwives: prevalence and association with burnout. *International Journal of Nursing Studies* 52(2): 578–87.

Simkin P. (1991) Just another day in a woman's life? Women's long-term perceptions of their first birth experience. *Part I. Birth* 18(4): 203–10.

Simpson M. and Catling C. (2015) *Understanding psychological traumatic birth experiences: A literature review. Women and Birth* 29(3): 203–7.

Sjoo M. (1973) Three Friends. *Spare Rib* 12: 19.

Sleep S., Grant A., Garcia J. and Chalmers I. (1984) West Berkshire perineal management trial. *British Medical Journal* 289: 587–90.

Smith J. (2002–2005) *The Shipman Enquiry – Reports 1–5.* CM 5853, 5854, 6249, 6934. The Shipman Enquiry, UK. http://webarchive.nationalarchives.gov.uk/20090808155110/ www.the-shipman-inquiry.org.uk/reports.asp (accessed 20 November 2017).

Smith J.A. and Osborn M. (2008) *Interpretive Phenomenological Analysis: A Practical Guide To Research Methods 2nd Edition.* London: Sage Publishing.

Stewart-Brown S.L., Platt S., Tennant A., Maheswaran H., Parkinson J., Weich S., Tennant R., Taggart F. and Clarke A. (2011) The Warwick-Edinburgh Mental Well-being Scale WEMWBS: a valid and reliable tool for measuring mental well-being in diverse populations and projects. *Journal of Epidemiology and Community Health* 65(2): A38–A39.

Tay S.L. (2006) *Activating the future: political documentaries and media activism. Afterimage: the journal of media arts and the cultural activism,* Vol. 34, nos. 1 & 2. 46–8.

Taylor M. (2010) The midwife as container. In Kirkham M. (ed.), *The Midwife-Mother Relationship 2nd Edition.* Basingstoke Hampshire: Palgrave Macmillan, 232-49.

The Journal.ie (2014) Taoiseach says Ireland is 'one of the safest places on the planet' to have a baby, 24 June. www.thejournal.ie/maternity-services-enda-kenny-1535382-Jun2014 (accessed 20 November 2017).

thelostboy (2011) The 25 Highest Grossing Documentaries of All Time. IndieWire. www.indiewire.com/2011/06/the-25-highest-grossing-documentaries-of-all-time-174232 (accessed 20 January 2017).

Tolofari M. (2014) Counting midwives. *Midwives* 17(1): 60–1.

TPM (2016) *Self-care and resilience in midwifery. The Practicing Midwife learning module.* www.practisingmidwife.co.uk/tpmindex.php?p1=curriculum&p2=module&p3=21 (accessed 13 July 2017).

Turpin J. (1986) The Dublin Society's Figure Drawing School and the Fine Arts in Dublin 1800–1849. *Dublin Historical Record* 39(2): 38–52.

Tyler I. and Baraitser L. (2013) Private View Public Birth: Making Feminist Sense of the New Visual Culture of Childbirth. *Studies in the Maternal* 5(2): 1–27. www.mamsie.bbk. ac.uk (accessed 20 November 2017).

UN (2015) *The Millennium Development Goal Report.* New York: United Nations. www.un.org/millenniumgoals/2015_MDG_Report/pdf/MDG%202015%20rev%20Jul y%201pdf (accessed August 2016).

Uvnäs-Moberg K., Handlin L and Petersson M (2015) Self-soothing behaviors with particular reference to oxytocin release induced by non-noxious sensory stimulation. *Frontiers in Psychology* 5:1529 (accessed 11 October 2017).

Wagner M. (1994) *Pursuing the Birth Machine: The Search for Appropriate Birth Technology.* Camperdown, Australia: ACE Graphics.

Walsh D. (2006) Subverting the assembly-line: childbirth in a free-standing birth centre. *Social Science & Medicine* 62(6): 1330–40.

Warwick C. (2016) Midwives can no longer keep services afloat. *Nursing Standard* 31(12): 27.

Warwick Medical School (2015). www2.warwick.ac.uk/fac/med/research/platform/wemwbs (accessed 12 July 2017).

Weber M. (1946) Bureaucracy. In H.H. Gerth and C. Wright Mills (eds), *From Max Weber: Essays in Sociology*. Oxford: Oxford University Press.

Werner E.R. and Korsch B.M. (1976) The vulnerability of the medical student: posthumous presentation of L.L. Stephens' ideas. *Pediatrics* 57(3): 321–328.

WHO (2008) *Millennium Development Goal 5 – improving maternal health: Improving Maternal Mental Health*. www.who.int/mental_health/prevention/suicide/Perinatal_depression_mmh_final.pdf (accessed August 2016).

WHO (2015) Caesarean sections should only be performed when medically necessary. Press release. www.who.int/mediacentre/news/releases/2015/caesarean-sections/en (accessed 20 November 2017).

Wickham S. (2014) Caring for ourselves. *The Practising Midwife* 17(11): 37–8.

Wickham S. (2015) *The most important thing women can do for themselves in the quest for a normal birth?* www.sarawickham.com (accessed 20 November 2017).

Wolin S. (1994) Fugitive Democracy. *Constellations* 1(1): 11–25.

Wood C. (2017) Report Review: The new Irish maternity strategy 2016–2026. *The Practising Midwife* 20(6): 33–5.

Your Dictionary (2017) Definition of 'hide-in-plain-sight'. www.yourdictionary.com/hidein-plain-sight#6VD5qJYgs0EBSBXd99 (accessed 15 July 2017).

INDEX